THE
NATURAL
PROSTATE CURE

YOUNG AGAIN PRODUCTS
310 N FRONT ST #150
WILMINGTON, NC 28401
(910) 371-2702 FAX ONLY
WWW.YOUNGAGAIN.COM
WWW.YOUNGAGAIN.ORG

Other Health Books
by Roger Mason

Lower Blood Pressure Without Drugs
The Minerals You Need
What Is Beta Glucan?
Lower Your Cholesterol Without Drugs
The Natural Diabetes Cure
No More Horse Estrogen!
Zen Macrobiotics for Americans
Testosterone Is Your Friend
The Supplements You Need

THE
NATURAL
PROSTATE CURE

A Practical Guide to
Using Diet and Supplements
for a Healthy Prostate

ROGER MASON

SQUAREONE
PUBLISHERS

The information and advice contained in this book are based upon the research and the personal and professional experiences of the author. They are not intended as a substitute for consulting with a healthcare professional. The publisher and author are not responsible for any adverse effects or consequences resulting from the use of any of the suggestions or procedures discussed in this book. All matters pertaining to your physical health should be supervised by a healthcare professional. It is a sign of wisdom, not cowardice, to seek a second or third opinion.

COVER DESIGNER: Jeannie Tudor
TYPESETTER: Theresa E. Wiscovitch

Square One Publishers
115 Herricks Road
Garden City Park, NY 11040
(516) 535-2010 • (877) 900-BOOK
www.squareonepublishers.com

Library of Congress Cataloging-in-Publication Data

Mason, Roger (Roger Wallace)
  The natural prostate cure : a practical guide to using diet and supplements for a healthy prostate / Roger Mason.—Rev. and updated.
      p. cm.
  Includes bibliographical references and index.
  ISBN 978-0-7570-0370-7 (pbk.)
  1. Prostate—Diseases--Alternative treatment. 2. Prostate—Diseases—Prevention.
3. Naturopathy. 4. Prostate--Popular works. I. Title.
  RC899.M37 2012
  616.99'463--dc23
                            2011040973

Contents

"If people let the government decide what foods they eat and what medicines they take, their bodies will soon be in as sorry a state as the souls who live under tyranny."

—THOMAS JEFFERSON

Introduction

In 2011 doctors are still castrating men and cutting their testicles off! This insanity has to stop. There is no reason for men to continue to be senselessly poisoned, irradiated, and butchered by the medical profession. Treating the symptoms, instead of the causes, of prostate disease has very drastic results—including diapers and impotence for the rest of a man's life. Prostate problems can be cured naturally with healthy diet, proven supplements, natural hormones, and fasting. *Diet and lifestyle cure disease.*

This book contains the distillation of forty years of prostate research. All of the information has been refined and written in plain English. This is the thirteenth time this book has been rewritten and expanded in the last nine years. This is the most informative, comprehensive, and researched book on prostate health in the world. Over two million men in most every country have now read *The Natural Prostate Cure.* By taking responsibility for their conditions, men can cure themselves naturally with the information herein.

The prostate is an integral part of the reproductive system, so any prostate-related illness can cause serious sexual performance problems. Men may encounter three main issues: infection (prostatitis), enlargement (benign prostate hypertrophy, or BPH), and cancer.

By the age of fifty, three out of four men already have enlarged prostates, and one in three men have cancer cells in their prostates. This, clearly, is not an "old man's disease" at all. By the time they reach the age of seventy-five, an astounding three out of four men in America have outright prostate cancer. It is the leading form of male cancer. The symptoms are very obvious—difficulty in urination, inability to empty the bladder completely, pain during sex or urination, sexual dysfunction, and, especially, the need to urinate in the middle of the night. All of these are classic symptoms of prostate problems.

The real cure comes from the results you bring about when you change your diet and lifestyle. Treat the very cause of your problem. Diet is everything. Natural health includes proper diet, proven supplements, natural hormone balance, weekly fasting, regular exercise, giving up prescription drugs, and ending negative habits (such as drinking coffee, overeating, consuming alcohol, and smoking). Holistic medicine treats the whole person instead of just alleviating the symptoms of a disease. Symptoms reflect the underlying causes of our illnesses and are harbingers of even worse health in the future. Always treat the cause of your illness and not just the symptoms.

1. Diet

Diet is everything! Diet cures disease. A wholesome, natural diet is the most important thing you need in order to get well and stay well. Diet and lifestyle cure illness. By eating a traditional wholegrain-based, low-fat diet, you can actually eliminate prostate infection, enlargement, and even cancer. If you doubt this, read actor Dirk Benedict's book *Confessions of a Kamikaze Cowboy*. Dirk was diagnosed with prostate cancer in his early thirties, and the doctors wanted to castrate him. That didn't appeal to him much, so he decided to go on a "macrobiotic" (Greek for overall view of life) diet of whole grains, beans, vegetables, soups, salads, seafood, and fruits. He quit eating red meat, poultry, eggs, dairy products, sweeteners of all kinds, refined foods, preservatives, and the like. After only seven months, Dirk knew he was well. He is now sixty-six, healthy, happy, youthful, vibrant, and the father of two grown sons. If Dirk had listened to his doctors, he would have died many years ago as a sexless eunuch in diapers.

Eating a natural diet of whole, unrefined low-fat foods is an essential part of getting well. Diet is everything. Supplements, hormones, exercise, and fasting are all secondary. When you are eating well, these additions are very powerful and make your recovery rapid. Without whole, healthy, natural food, it doesn't matter what else you do; you're just not going to get well. *Diet cures disease.*

THE SECRET TO GOOD HEALTH

We've all heard of people, like the Okinawans for example, who live very long lives and have low disease rates. Well, you don't have to live in a remote farming village and give up all the conveniences of the modern world to live a long and healthy life. You just have to change your diet and lifestyle. Such long-lived people eat whole grains, beans, vegetables, seafood, local fruits, and very little, if any, meat, poultry, eggs, or dairy products. Generally, their fat intake makes up only about 10 percent of their diet and consists of mainly vegetable oils, rather than saturated animal fats.

Most of the current diet authors give terrible advice on how to eat. Their personal health proves this. There are only a few who really have any idea what they're doing and actually practice what they preach. Gary Null, Robert Pritikin, Neal Barnard, Terry Shintani, Susan Powter, Dean Ornish, and a very few others write reasonable books on eating well. Any of the authors of macrobiotic books, such as Michio Kushi, are better. For optimum health, your diet should be based on whole grains and beans. Whole grains are the staff of life. Most all vegetables are fine, but the nightshade family (potatoes, tomatoes, peppers, eggplant) should be avoided. Also avoid vegetables containing excess oxalic acid (spinach, rhubarb, red chard). Any bean or legume is fine, and there are dozens of varieties. Beans are good food. Local fruit can be eaten in moderation. Seafood can also be eaten in moderation if you do not want to be a vegetarian, as long as you are not allergic to it. Nuts are very high in fat (90 percent fat calories generally) and should only be used as a garnish. Soups and salads are good additions to your meals if they are made with macrobiotic ingredients. Avoid red meat, poultry, eggs, and dairy products of all kinds. Do not eat refined foods, processed foods, or sweeteners of any kind (including honey). Steer clear of tropical foods such as citrus, pineapples, mangos, and coconuts (all of which are meant for tropical populations in their native environments). Tropical races living in warm climates can and should eat such foods, of course.

One of the best studies on prostate health was conducted at Loma Linda University (the *American Journal of Epidemiology* v 120, 1982). Researchers studied 6,735 men for what they ate. The men had a direct relation between the animal foods they ate and their rates of prostate cancer. (They also had the same direct relation with obesity.) The more meat or poultry they ate, the more cancer they got. The more milk and cheese they ate, the more cancer they got. The more eggs they ate, the more cancer they got. The really interesting thing about these findings is that men who ate meat, poultry, eggs, *and* cheese had extremely high prostate cancer rates. These foods work synergistically to support malignancies. This study, among others, proves the basic thesis that an excess of dietary saturated animal fat is the underlying cause of prostate disease. As you will see in the next chapter, an abundance of statistical data strongly supports this theory.

THE STAFF OF LIFE

Whole grains are the basis of your daily food. This includes brown rice, whole grain breads, whole wheat pasta, corn, barley, rye, millet, oats, spelt, buckwheat, and quinoa. People who eat whole grains are healthier, live longer, and are less likely to develop diseases of all kinds. Americans only eat about 1 percent whole grains when they should be eating at least 50 percent. The fact that we eat a mere 1 percent of whole grains says everything about our diet. At the University of California in San Diego (*Integrative Cancer Therapies* v 5, 2006), progressive doctors gave prostate cancer patients a low-fat, wholegrain-based diet including lots of vegetables for six months. These men improved remarkably and lived longer than the patients receiving the standard medical treatment. At the University of California in Los Angeles (the *American Journal of Clinical Nutrition* v 86, 2007), men were put on a vegetarian form of the Pritikin diet. Their insulin levels fell dramatically, and their risk factors for prostate cancer were greatly reduced. Again at the University of California in Los Angeles (*Recent Results in Cancer Research* v 166, 2005), studies showed that metabolic syndrome (high blood sugar and insulin resistance) correlated with prostate cancer. Men given a low-fat diet and exercise lowered their insulin levels greatly. At Queen's University in Canada (the *International Journal of Cancer* v 116, 2005), doctors studied the dietary patterns of men. Those who included whole grains and vegetables in their daily fare had far lower prostate cancer rates than the ones who ate meat, milk, sugar, and refined grains. Dean Ornish's Preventive Medicine Research Institute (the *Journal of the American Dietetic Association* v 105, 2005) has been working with prostate cancer patients. They gave these patients a low-fat vegan diet with very impressive results: The patients lived longer and had much better health. Dean and his associates at the University of California in San Francisco (the *Journal of Urology* v 174, 2005) fed prostate cancer patients a vegan diet for one year. Patients also took a few basic supplements and exercised regularly. The men refused all traditional medical treatments including surgery, drugs, and radiation. This simple regimen slowed down, and even reversed, the cancer growth. If Dean would just go a little further and adopt macrobiotics, proven supplements, natural hormones, and fasting, these men could be cured of cancer instead of just living longer. An entire book, *Whole Grain Foods in Health and Disease* (2002), edited by Marquart et al., is devoted to the health benefits of eating whole, unprocessed, unrefined grains. The authors found that people who eat whole grains are far less likely to get cancer, especially prostate or breast cancer.

Americans eat very few fresh (or frozen) green and yellow vegetables. Asians in general eat the most vegetables and prepare them in the most delicious ways; they also tend to consume a

The Power of Soy

Soy foods are very effective in reducing the rates of various cancers, especially prostate and breast cancer. Asian cultures eat quite a lot of these soy foods in various forms. The longest-lived people on earth, the Okinawans, eat more than anyone with a soy intake of 12 percent. It is unrealistic and impractical to ask westerners to do this for several reasons. Soybeans per se, just don't taste very good. Tofu is not a whole food; nor is it very nutritious. Most people have never heard of tempeh, seitan, or annatto and have little interest in eating them. Soy sauce is merely a condiment. A little miso goes a long way, but it is basically used only in soup. How much soy flour can you really add to your baked goods? Soy milk is rather high in calories (about 120 per cup) and should be limited to cooking rather than used as a beverage. Soy isoflavones, as a supplement, are really the most practical way to use soy and are recommended in Chapter 3.

great deal of soy products (refer to the above inset on "The Power of Soy" to learn how soy can be especially helpful in reducing prostate cancer rates). You want to eat more fresh (or even frozen vegetables, since they actually have more nutrients) every day. Johns Hopkins University (the *American Journal of Clinical Nutrition* v 85, 2007) studied over 30,000 men. They found a strong correlation between the large amount of vegetables the men ate and the small number of men who developed prostate disease. At the Negri Institute in Italy, doctors found the same phenomenon (the *International Journal of Cancer* v 109, 2004). Vegetables and vegetable fiber protected men from prostate cancer.

CUTTING OUT FAT

Meat, poultry, eggs, and dairy contain heavy amounts of saturated fat, which is the main dietary cause of prostate and other cancers. *Saturated animal fat is the basic cause of prostate disease.* Vegetable oils should only be used in moderation at 10 to 20 percent total calories, since they have not been correlated per se with prostate cancer. At Wake Forest University (*Prostate* v 63, 2005), it was found that the phytanic acid found in red meat and dairy products definitely contributes to cancer of the prostate. "Phytanic acid, which primarily comes from dietary intake of dairy and red meat may be associated with prostate cancer risk." The National Cancer Institute studied the diets of 29,361 men (*Cancer Research* v 65, 2005) and showed that red meat is definitely a prostate cancer promoter. In general, animal foods promote disease.

Dairy milk (including low-fat milk) contains large amounts of lactose and casein, regardless of the fat content. The protein casein has been shown to promote cancer. Drinking milk has repeatedly been shown to correlate with prostate disease (*Prostate* v 33, 1997 and *Science* v 285, 1999). Yogurt actually has twice the amount of lactose, since dried milk powder is added to thicken it. People of all races, especially blacks and Asians, lose their ability to digest lactose after the age of three (when humans no longer produce lactase, the enzyme necessary to digest dairy). Adding lactase tablets to your dairy foods or buying lactose-reduced milk will not solve the problem. Visit the Internet Web site NotMilk.com to learn more. Instead, use soy, almond, oat, or rice milk, whether refrigerated or in aseptic shelf packs, as these items are now commonly available in grocery stores. Take dairy out of your life.

The proof is overwhelming: Dairy intake causes prostate disease. At the Fox Chase Cancer Center (the *American Journal Clinical Nutrition* v 81, 2005), "Dairy intake may increase prostate cancer risk." At the National Institute of Health (the *International Journal of Cancer* v 120, 2007), "Total dairy intake was also positively associated with risk of prostate cancer." At Inserm in Paris (the *British Journal of Nutrition* v 95, 2006), "Our data support the hypothesis that dairy products have a harmful effect with respect to the risk of prostate cancer." At the University of Bristol (the *British Journal of Cancer* v 88, 2003), they found intake of dairy foods raised IGF-1 (insulin-like growth factor 1) levels, which in turn raised the rates of prostate, breast, and other cancers.

CUTTING OUT SUGAR

Insulin resistance (high insulin and blood sugar levels) has been correlated with prostate disease. Americans eat about 160 pounds of various unneeded sweeteners in their food every year. Asians and Africans, who have the lowest prostate disease rates, eat only a fraction of that amount. Excess sugar consumption of any kind can cause hyperinsulinemia (the presence of excess insulin in the blood), insulin resistance, high blood sugar, and diabetes. Blood sugar dysmetabolism and metabolic syndrome (pre-diabetes) are two causes of insulin disease. *Sugar is sugar is sugar*, whether it is honey, maple syrup, brown sugar, "raw" sugar, molasses, sorghum syrup, cane syrup, dextrose, fructose, maltose, fruit syrup, amazake, fruit juice, fruit concentrate, invert sugar, corn syrup, agave, dried fruit, or any other form of sweetener. This includes stevia, sucralose, and other sugar substitutes, since they act like sugar in our bodies. It's always good for a laugh to see someone in a health food store paying several dollars for a small bag of "raw" sugar or agave nectar, thinking that this is somehow different, not really sugar, and not really bad for them.

ENDING BAD HABITS

Bad habits such as smoking, drinking alcohol, using recreational drugs, and drinking coffee obviously worsen your health. Smoking ages people dramatically. Smoking is clearly correlated with prostate cancer. More than one drink of alcohol a day causes poor health in general. Coffee, along with caffeinated energy drinks, is an epidemic addiction. The use of various recreational drugs, addictive or not, is also epidemic. Lack of exercise is another basic cause of bad health overall. Obesity is definitely correlated with prostate conditions (*Urology* v 58, 2001). Being overweight strongly increases your chances of getting prostate disease. Exercise is vital for good health, especially if you are trying to recover from an illness. Study after study shows how being overweight causes higher rates of every known illness (except osteoporosis). Does anything correlate *positively* with prostate health? Yes, whole grains, fiber, and vegetable intake do, as do slimness, eating fewer calories, and low-fat diets.

LESS IS MORE

It is very important to eat fewer calories. Americans eat about twice the calories, twice the protein, and more than five times the fat they need. Yes, we eat for two people. *Calorie restriction is the most proven and effective way to extend your life span.* Nothing else has been shown to make you live longer and live better than eating fewer calories. Long-term clinical studies with animals, including monkeys, have proven this fact; moreover, short-term human studies also have verified the benefits of eating fewer calories. The only author on this subject is Roy Walford, who wrote *The 120-Year Diet* and *Maximum Lifespan*. (Unfortunately, he went in a different direction with *Beyond the 120-Year Diet*.)

The average man needs only about 1,800 calories a day, and a woman only needs about 1,200 calories. You can easily eat just two meals a day, instead of three. You can also fast (fasting means *only* consuming water) one day a week by skipping breakfast and lunch on a specified day. Just eat dinner on a given night and don't eat again until dinner the next night. Longer fasts may be done periodically for more powerful effects. Doctors at the University of Wisconsin (*Prostate* v 36, 1998) improved the immunity of prostate glands in rats by merely lowering their calorie intake. Other doctors at the university showed that lowering the calorie intake of mice altered their entire genetic aging profile and allowed them to live much longer, with greatly enhanced immunity. Researchers in Takatsuki, Japan (*Takeda Kenkyushoho* v 53, 1994) actually reduced the prostate weights of rats by simply giving them less food. Doctors at the University of Umea in Sweden (the Journal of Cancer v 58, 1986) gave rats with prostate cancer less food, inhibiting the growth of their tumors. Long-term studies on primates about calorie restriction have shown excellent results. At the Hutchison Cancer Center (*Cancer Epidemiology* v 11, 2002), men who ate the least calories had only half the prostate cancer of the control group. This, in addition to eating the right foods, is the most effective means you can use to lengthen and improve the quality of your life.

CONCLUSION

Not long ago, the Atkins, Paleolithic, and "ketogenic" diets were popular, until obese and sickly Robert Atkins fell over dead. The awful South Beach Diet followed and went by the wayside as well. This has been replaced by the irrational and ineffective "glycemic index." Diets such as these favor unlimited meat, dairy, and fat, yet avoid whole grains! Whole grains should be the very basis of your diet. Ketosis is, in fact, a pathological state in which the body is literally starving for complex carbohydrates. The "glycemic index" classifies whole grains, such as brown rice and oatmeal, as being identical in effect to simple sugars such as cake or candy. The standard of reference is white bread! This is completely asinine. Start using brown rice instead of white rice or potatoes. Eat whole wheat pasta instead of refined white pasta. Find 100 percent whole grain breads without preservatives. Buy 100 percent whole grain hot and cold cereals without sugar. *Make whole grains the basis of each meal.* The words "carbohydrates" or "carbs" are basically meaningless. Eating simple sugars and refined grains should certainly be avoided. Whole grains are literally the "staff of life," and always have been throughout history. Whole grains have been our staple food since mankind first learned to cultivate crops and became independent. Make whole grains and beans the very basis of your daily food.

2. Fats

Fatty foods of all kinds, especially saturated animal fats like red meat, poultry, eggs, and dairy products, seem to hold a hypnotic attraction for many people. Studies for the last fifty years have proven repeatedly that high-fat diets cause disease, poor health, and early death. Deep inside, we all know that high-fat diets are bad for us. They cause obesity, clog our arteries, promote various cancers, and shorten our lives. Americans eat 42 percent fat calories! Most all of these are saturated animal fats, which are the most harmful. Fortunately, the Atkins or ketogenic diet has faded, but it's been replaced with the ridiculous glycemic index. This emphasizes animal foods over whole grains and beans since fats and proteins cause almost no blood sugar response. Eating all the meat, poultry, eggs, and dairy products you want is obviously the road to Hell. It seems that people just want an excuse to do what they want to do, while endlessly rationalizing bad habits. In America, and in most European countries, the diet is about 40 percent fats, most of which are the saturated animal kind. The more affluent a society is, the richer the diet is in animal foods and saturated fats—and the higher the disease rates. Ironically, prosperity brings poor health.

HIGH FAT INTAKE AND PROSTATE DISEASE

Study after study shows that high fat intake is correlated with every disease known. This is not debatable. Any diet guru who tells you to eat meat, poultry, eggs, or dairy products is a *prima facie* fraud. High fat intake is especially correlated with prostate disease and prostate cancer. There are just too many studies to list that show the relation of fat intake, especially saturated animal fat, to prostate disease. Please take a long look at Figure 2.1 on page 15; it will leave no doubt in your mind that *saturated fat intake is the major cause of prostate cancer-related deaths.* The figure is based on the diets of literally billions of people and just cannot be contested. The diets of men in countries like China and Japan get only about 10 percent of their calories from fat. These people suffer only a fraction of the prostate cancer-related deaths that we have in America. If 20 men per 100,000 die from prostate cancer in the United States, fewer than 5 men per 100,000 die in China. Point made.

THE TRUTH ABOUT FAT

Hydrogenated fats are the worst, as they do not exist in nature. These fats are made in laboratories with hydrogen gas, extreme pressures, and platinum catalysts. Our bodies simply cannot deal with this artificial, synthetic fat, which ends up clogging our arteries. Eating vegetable oils is simply a lesser evil. The idea that there are "good fats" and "bad fats" is an illusion. Olive oil intake, for example, should be as limited as any other fat intake. The less fat you eat, the better! The less fat you eat, the healthier you will be and the longer you will live. When Asian or African men move to the United States but maintain their traditional diets, they still get almost no prostate disease of any kind. This is called a "migration study," and the results are inarguable.

Mediterranean countries that consume olive oil rather than butter do have slightly lower prostate disease rates than other European countries, but these rates are still much higher than those of Asian countries. The only exception to the fat "rule" is when a supplement of 1–2 g per day of flaxseed oil is taken. Flax is a much better choice than fish oil for a lot of reasons. Flax oil

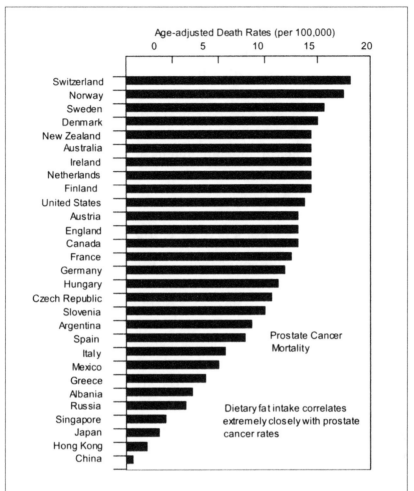

FIGURE 2.1. Prostate cancer mortality rates. This figure compares the prostate cancer-related death rates per 100,000 people in twenty-nine countries. Note that the people of China, who traditionally eat a very low-fat diet, have the lowest number of prostate-related deaths.

contains valuable omega-3 fatty acids, at a mere nine calories per gram—an insignificant daily calorie intake. Our dietary ratio of omega-6 fatty acids to omega-3s is too high. We eat few foods that contain the omega-3s. Buy and keep your flax oil refrigerated.

Nuts can be eaten in moderation as a garnish. Nuts are usually about 90 percent fat calories, so they cannot be used as a main source of food. Toasted nuts add lots of flavor to your basic foods. Peanuts are tropical legumes and one of the top ten allergenic foods known. Eat temperate nuts like almonds, walnuts, pine nuts, and pecans, rather than tropical ones like cashews and Brazil nuts (though people native to tropical areas certainly can eat these). There is no botanical category "tree nuts," as every one is completely different in species and unrelated to any others. The concept of "tree nut allergies" is *prima facie* ridiculous, and food labels that state such things are meaningless. Peanuts are the real allergen.

THE PROOF IS IN YOUR FAT

The American Health Foundation, in Valhalla, New York, has done a fine job of showing how a low-fat, high-fiber diet slows the development of prostate cancer. Native South African black men have extremely low prostate disease rates on their traditional diets. When fed a typical American high-fat diet, their testosterone levels fell, their estrogen levels rose (and thus, their testosterone-to-estrogen ratio worsened), and they got more prostate disease (*Bulletin of the New York Academy of Medicine* v 56, 1980 and *Cancer Research* v 42, 1982).

Again, the American Health Foundation carried out an in-depth review of the scientific studies to show that omega-6 fatty acids stimulate prostate cancer growth, while omega-3 fatty acids (like flax oil) inhibit it (the *Journal of the National Cancer Institute* v 85, 1993). The problem is that the omega-3s are rare in foods, while omega-6s are all too common. Red meat contains arachidonic acid, which is generally nonexistent in plant foods. This is considered to be the single most dangerous fatty acid known, and it is a precursor of the inflammatory chemical prostaglandin E_2. More reason not to eat meat. Harvard Medical School presented similar findings regarding the relationship between omega-6 fatty acids and prostate cancer, as well as a long list of other diseases that are clearly associated with fat intake. Studies continue at the University of Tokyo, University of Wales, University of Michigan, National Cancer Institute, University of Ohio, and many other clinics around the world. All have come to the same conclusion that dietary saturated fat causes prostate disease. Just some of the many studies can be found in:

❏ *American Journal of Clinical Nutrition* v 66, 1997.

❏ *Annual Review of Nutrition* v 18, 1998.

❏ *Anticancer Research* v 16, 1996.

❏ *British Journal of Urology* v 77, 1996.

❏ *Cancer Epidemiology Biomarkers Preview* v 5, 1996.

❏ *Cancer Research* v 54, 1994.

❏ *Journal of the National Cancer Institute* v 85, 1993.

❏ *Lipids* v 27, 1992.

❏ *Nutrition Research* v 14, 1994.

❏ *Proceedings of the Society for Experimental and Biological Medicine* v 216, 1997.

The study in *Lipids* (v 27, 1992), for example, is from the American Health Foundation. They clearly state, "International comparisons suggest a relationship between prostate cancer incidence and dietary fat, an inference supported by migration studies. N-6 [or omega-6] fatty acids stimulate and N-3 [omega-3] fatty acids inhibit human prostate cells." They then present overwhelming evidence from around the world to support these findings.

CONCLUSION

It is quite obvious that fat intake, especially from animal fat, is the biggest factor in prostate disease. The more fats you eat, especially saturated fats, the more chance you have of getting prostate cancer, BPH, and prostatitis. Would you rather eat red meat and dairy products, and die a painful, lingering, premature death; or would you rather change your diet and live a healthier, happier, longer life? Eating fat raises your estradiol and estrone levels, causes all manner of illness, and makes you obese. This is the main reason American and European men over the age of fifty have higher estrogen levels than women of the same age! That's right, western men over fifty generally have more estrogen (estradiol and estrone) in their blood than their wives do after menopause! This is frightening!

Fat intake also increases the levels of harmful "free radicals" in our bodies. Free radicals are molecules with unpaired electrons, and they damage our health by attacking healthy cells in an attempt to balance the electrical charge they carry. Referred to as "oxidative damage," this effect not only harms our metabolism but also shortens our life span. Oxidative damage is a major factor in aging, but by making better food choices, you can lower the amount of free radicals in your body and live a longer, healthier life.

The ideal diet contains only 10 percent fat calories from vegetables (or even seafood). The maximum is 20 percent fat calories, mostly from vegetables. Eating any more fat than this will simply not benefit you. You must eat less than one-fifth of your calories as fats and oils, and no more than that. Lowering fat intake from 40 percent fat calories to say 25 percent just won't do anything at all. To benefit from a low-fat diet, you must eat less than 20 percent fat calories, preferably about 10 percent. Pseudoscientific "studies" will lower fat calorie intake to around 30 percent, and then claim there were no benefits found—no wonder! Achieving good health is not difficult to do when you simply make better food choices. Taking red meat, poultry, eggs, and dairy out of your daily fare will basically solve the problem.

3. Supplements

Always remember that continually making better food choices is the most important thing we can do for our health. Natural health is about diet and lifestyle. Lifestyle factors include exercise, stress, smoking, alcohol intake, prescription and recreational drug use, and even coffee consumption. Supplements are important but very secondary to diet. You receive far, far more health benefits with both proper diet *and* supplements than with diet alone. All of the supplements discussed in this chapter are natural, safe, and inexpensive. They all have numerous clinical studies behind them that show their value to prostate health and to health in general. This chapter is not going to use extensive references; however, please realize that all of these supplements have been proven effective after four decades of scientific research including various clinical studies.

SUPPLEMENTS FOR PROSTATE HEALTH

A number of dietary supplements have shown potential in the treatment of prostate disease. Some of the most promising are beta-sitosterol, flaxseed oil, soy isoflavones, and vitamin D. A discussion of each of these supplements, as well as several others, follows.

Beta-carotene

Beta-carotene is a powerful, proven, and well-known antioxidant. A study published in *Cancer Research* showed that the intake of beta-carotene had a strong correlation with reduced prostate cancer in Japanese men. Many other studies have shown similar results. Supplementing your diet with beta-carotene is better than taking vitamin A because beta-carotene is a precursor to vitamin A, so you won't overload your body, even with higher doses.

DOSAGE: Beta-carotene is an important antioxidant with many health benefits, so take 10,000 IU daily (any brand is fine).

Beta-sitosterol

Sterols are plant alcohols that occur in every vegetable you eat. Clinical studies over the last thirty years have shown that beta-sitosterol is the most important supplement for good prostate (and cholesterol) health. The studies on beta-sitosterol are listed in Chapter 5. It's very important you understand that herbal products such as saw palmetto, pygeum, nettles, etc., contain almost no (generally one-thirtieth of 1 percent) beta-sitosterol, even though it is the active ingredient. These products are of no

---

Supplement Measurements: IU vs. MG

Finding the right supplements to complete your diet can be difficult, especially with so many different products on the market. An important detail to keep in mind is how different supplements are measured. Some supplements are measured in international units (IU) while others are calculated per milligram (mg). International units measure the strength or potency of a substance while milligrams measure its weight.

value. Analytical testing has shown that there are simply no biologically significant amounts of beta-sitosterol—even in the most expensive extracts. To prove this to yourself, just read the label; you will not find beta-sitosterol listed, and there are no other active ingredients! There are no human tests that suggest these products are actually effective.

DOSAGE: Take 300 mg to 600 mg of mixed sterols a day. Make sure the label says at least 300 mg of mixed plant sterols.

Coenzyme Q$_{10}$

Coenzyme Q$_{10}$, or CoQ$_{10}$, is a powerful enzyme in our bodies, but our CoQ$_{10}$ levels fall as we age. Studies have shown that CoQ$_{10}$ helps prevent and cure various forms of cancer as well as other diseases. At Nagoya University in Japan, scientists found that when CoQ$_{10}$ was added to cells taken from BPH patients, it had a very beneficial effect on their metabolism. CoQ$_{10}$ has amazing health benefits for our heart, brain, kidneys, liver, and other organs. Everyone over forty should take this supplement.

DOSAGE: You must take at least 100 mg of CoQ$_{10}$ daily. If you are sickly, or have cancer, take 200 mg daily for one year. Be sure to take at least 100 mg a day of real Japanese ubiquinone (CoQ$_{10}$), even though most brands offer much less than 100 mg. The price of real Japanese CoQ$_{10}$ is as low as twenty dollars for sixty capsules. Do *not* take ubiquinol as it is unstable and has no shelf life. The label *must* say Japanese ubiquinone.

Flaxseed Oil

Flaxseed oil is very good for prostate health and the best known source of omega-3 fatty acids. Consuming 1,000–2,000 mg ($^1/_2$ teaspoon) of omega-3 fatty acids daily is good for people of all ages. Two articles in *Anticancer Research* showed that omega-3 fatty acids have important protective properties for human prostate cells in vitro. "The Health Professionals Follow-up Study," which analyzed the diets of 51,529 men, showed that omega-6 fatty acids were positively associated with prostate cancer rates. Omega-3 fatty acids, on the other hand, were associated with prostate health. In Beijing, researchers at Peking Medical College gave men flax extract for four months, which dramatically increased their urine flow as well as their International Prostate Symptom Score (or IPSS, which is based on a questionnaire made up of various important diagnostic factors, and is the most accepted diagnostic measurement of prostate health). A study involving prostate cancer patients was done at Duke University. Men given a flax supplement slowed down their cancer growth in only thirty-four days. When self-appointed Internet authorities tell you that flax oil is bad for prostate health, now you'll know they walk in darkness. The more research done on omega-3s and flaxseed oil, the more health benefits are revealed.

Flaxseed is by far the best source of omega-3 fatty acids. Flax oil supplements are preferable to fish liver oil supplements for many reasons. Flax has more omega-3s and is less subject to rancidity. The many studies on omega-3 fatty acids that used fish liver oils are equally applicable to flax oil. There are many good reasons to take flax oil daily, but it is especially beneficial for cardiovascular health.

DOSAGE: Just 2,000 mg a day of flax oil is very beneficial and only 18 calories. When you buy flax oil, make sure it has been refrigerated, and keep it refrigerated to prevent oxidation.

Glutathione

Glutathione is one of our four basic antioxidant enzymes, and it is a critical part of our immune system. Glutathione levels are important for prostate health, but blood and tissue glutathione levels typically fall as people age. Taking glutathione alone is expensive, not to mention somewhat ineffective. Fortunately, you can take an inexpensive 600 mg capsule of N-acetyl cysteine, or NAC, to enhance your glutathione levels very effectively and safely. In the last few years, there has been quite a bit of good research published on the value of NAC supplements. By maintaining a youthful glutathione level, you will gain many health benefits; in particular, boosting your glutathione levels will improve your immune system, so you can better resist disease.

DOSAGE: Take 600 mg of NAC daily. NAC is widely available, so buy any good brand.

Minerals

Minerals are essential for prostate health, and we are woefully mineral deficient. No matter how well you eat, you just aren't going to get all the minerals you need because our farm and crop soils are in such poor condition and lacking in so many elements. Minerals work synergistically, so you need all of them to be healthy. We have only begun to study the importance of minerals on prostate function, but it is already clear that you will never have good prostate health as long as you are mineral deficient. Find a mineral supplement that contains the required amounts of all twenty known elements our bodies need. (Actually, our bodies need twenty-four minerals, but we get enough sodium, potassium, sulfur, and phosphorous in our diets already.) This includes boron, calcium, chromium, cobalt, copper, germanium, iodine, iron, magnesium, manganese, molybdenum, gallium, cesium, nickel, selenium, silicon, strontium, tin, vanadium, and zinc. The two most important minerals for prostate health are selenium and zinc. However, the point is to get all the minerals you need, and not just the two most important. The multivitamin and mineral supplements you see generally have only about ten of these elements. Look for a mineral-only supplement that contains at least these twenty vital minerals in the amounts you need. Try searching the Internet for "mineral supplements." You do *not* need to supplement sodium, potassium, sulfur, or phosphorous. Avoid colloidal minerals (extremely small mineral particles that remain suspended in liquid rather than dissolving) and coral calcium, as these do not contain any biologically significant mineral amounts. *Read the label* to see which minerals are included, and in what amounts. It is important to realize that we need all of the known minerals. In the future, science will probably show that we need other minerals such as barium, rubidium, europium, neodymium, praseodymium, thulium, lithium, samarium, tungsten, lanthanum, and yttrium. Barium is a regular trace element and we take in about 1,000 mcg daily. Rubidium is also a regular trace element and we take in about 1,000 mcg of that as well. There are definitely ultra-trace elements that will eventually prove to be vital. These include those minerals listed above as well as several others, which will be discussed further in Chapter 4.

DOSAGE: To learn the optimal daily intake for each of these vital minerals, refer to Table 3.1 on pages 37 and 38. This table provides you with the appropriate doses of all twenty minerals. In the following chapter, each mineral is discussed in detail, so you can learn the specific benefits, and in some cases, the drawbacks of these essential nutrients.

Quercetin

Quercetin is a potent and proven plant-derived antioxidant, but it is not yet well known. You will hear more about this effective supplement. Studies in the *Journal of Steroid Biochemistry, Urology,* and the Japanese journal *Daizu Tanpakushitsu Kenkyukai Kaishi* show that quercetin can help promote prostate health. A new study at the Mayo Clinic, published in *Carcinogenesis,* suggests that quercetin may have real value in fighting against prostate cancer. Quercetin is a beneficial supplement for many other reasons besides being an excellent antioxidant, but since it just isn't found in most common foods, it is a borderline endogenous supplement (an endogenous supplement would be one that is produced in our bodies and/or found in our everyday diet).

DOSAGE: A daily dosage of 100 mg of any brand is good, as a normal diet only provides about 10 mg (mostly from apples and onions).

Soy Isoflavones

Soy isoflavones have finally seen a lot of research regarding their health benefits. Studies have shown that these isoflavones have great health benefits for your prostate. The main components in soy that we are concerned with are genistein and daidzein. These are flavones (plant pigments) and unrelated to hormones or prohormones (precursors to hormones). Genistein and daidzein are not "phytoestrogens." There is no estrogen, or any other hormone—testosterone, progesterone, dehydroepiandrosterone (DHEA), melatonin, etc.—in plants. Soy does not have estrogenic effects. *There is no such thing as a phytoestrogen!*

Studies on soy benefits for prostate health have been published in journals such as *Prostate, Anticancer Research*, the *Journal of Endocrinology, Nutrition and Cancer*, the *Journal of Steroid Biochemistry, Cancer Epidemiology, Biomarkers & Prevention*, the *American Journal of Clinical Nutrition, Cancer Letters*, the *International Journal of Oncology*, and many others. The proof here is overwhelming. You may see Internet sites warning against the "dangers" of soy, but this is simply propaganda from the dairy and meat industries (especially the Weston Price Foundation).

DOSAGE: A good brand of soy isoflavones will list the amount of genistein and daidzein on the label. Take a total of 40 mg daily. Soy foods, especially refined foods such as tofu, generally are an impractical source of isoflavones. Soy isoflavone supplements are a much more practical and realistic means of isoflavone intake.

Vitamin D

Vitamin D deficiency is epidemic. Vitamin D does not occur in our food in any meaningful amount. Vitamin D_3 is really a hormone that is produced in our bodies when we are exposed to sunlight. *This is the most important "vitamin" for your prostate.* Most of the research on vitamin D and the prostate has been done only in the last ten years. There are hundreds of clinical studies demonstrating the importance of vitamin D in prostate function. These include studies in such journals as *Cancer Research, Anticancer Research, Prostate, Clinical Cancer Research, Cancer Letters, Surgical Forum,* and other respected international publications. One study at Stanford University, which treated men with prostate cancer with no other therapy than vitamin D_3 supplements, had very impressive results.

DOSAGE: Take 800 IU of vitamin D a day (unless you're out in the sun regularly); this is a safe amount, especially in wintertime when we get little exposure to the sun. Vitamin D_3 is fat-soluble, so don't listen to "experts" who tell you to take more than 800 IU a day. Sickly or elderly people, however, can take up to 1,200 IU.

Vitamin E

Vitamin E is a very beneficial nutrient, especially for our cardiovascular health. Our American diets are generally very deficient in vitamin E. Whole grains are the best source of vitamin E, but most of us eat only 1 percent whole grains a day. This is the second-most important vitamin for your prostate. There are countless published studies from around the world that show the value of vitamin E supplementation for prostate health, and for health in general. Every year more studies are published. Vitamin E is a basic and proven supplement for people of all ages, but many other vitamins are also essential to our health. The inset on page 27 provides more information on vitamins.

DOSAGE: Your daily vitamin pill will contain the Reference Daily Intake (RDI) of vitamin E, but that's only 30 IU. Supplement your diet with 200 IU daily of mixed natural tocopherols, and note that this is seven times the RDI. Or take a 400 IU capsule every other day. Be careful not to take too much because overdoses will thin your blood. And don't use the cheap brands that contain only d-alpha tocopherol.

OTHER NUTRIENTS TO CONSIDER

Too often our diets lack the proper nutrients, but there are so many supplements on the market that it is difficult to determine the best products for your body. The following list of supplements may not have any specific value in curing prostate disease, but they offer many other important health benefits.

Acetyl-L-carnitine

Acetyl-L-carnitine, or ALC, is simply the acetyl derivative of regular carnitine, which is found mainly in red meat. ALC is more easily absorbed than carnitine, but no matter how good your diet is, your ALC levels will fall as you age. The most important benefit of ALC is that it is good for brain metabolism and memory. ALC also supports cognition, learning, clear thinking, sound sleep, nerve transmission and other neuroprotective benefits.

Vitamins

Vitamins are important. There are only thirteen vitamins, and there is an RDI set for each. Be especially careful when you are selecting vitamin B and vitamin C supplements. Be sure to find a multivitamin with 1 mg of methylcobalamin instead of regular cobalamin (vitamin B_{12}); vitamin B_{12} is just not orally absorbed. Vitamin C, on the other hand, can be absorbed orally. We only need about 60 mg a day of vitamin C, and that is supplied in our daily food. Taking more than 250 mg a day of vitamin C is harmful and will, over time, acidify your blood (which is naturally alkaline, having a pH level of 7.4), causing numerous side effects. Megadoses of any nutrient unbalance the body's metabolism. *Do not take more than 250 mg of vitamin C a day.* There is really no reason to take a vitamin C supplement other than what is in your daily vitamin tablet. For all other vitamins, simply take the recommended daily intake.

DOSAGE: Take 500 to 1,000 mg of ALC a day. Use this with phosphatidyl serine (PS) and pregnenolone, which you learn about later on, for synergistic results.

Acidophilus

Acidophilus, and other probiotics, shows no specific benefit for prostate health per se, but it is important to add this to your supplements list. Our bodies work as a holistic system, and our digestion is obviously vital to our total health. *Good health begins with our digestion.* Our digestive tracts are generally in terrible shape from overeating and from eating the wrong foods. Consuming whole, healthy foods, eating lower calorie foods, fasting one day a week, and taking a good brand of acidophilus daily can improve your entire digestive system.

DOSAGE: A good brand of acidophilus should state that every capsule has at least six billion live multi-strain organisms and eight strains at the time of manufacture. Do not be misled by "per gram" counts rather than per capsule. Buy it, and keep it refrigerated. You can also find the spore form of acidophilus, called "lacto spore," that does not require refrigeration; this can be taken in addition to regular acidophilus if you like.

Beta Glucan

Beta glucan is the most potent immune system-enhancing supplement known to science. It has been studied for its power against tumors and cancer. It doesn't matter whether beta glucan comes from yeast and mushrooms (1,3/1,6 configuration) or oats and barley (1,3/1,4 configuration). All 1,3 configurations of true beta glucan polysaccharides have the same potency. Beta glucan has proven power to stimulate our immune system. With its amazing ability to fight infections and ward off illnesses, the power of beta glucan has been known for over twenty-five years now. This is definitely a supplement people of all ages need to take. Yet only in the last few years have advances in technology allowed us to extract it easily and inexpensively. Currently, yeast is the least expensive source of beta glucan.

DOSAGE: Economical 200 mg supplements are available for about ten dollars for sixty capsules. Still, there is a lot of advertising misinformation about beta glucan, especially on the Internet, so be careful when selecting the right brand for you.

Carnosine

Carnosine is a very important supplement because it is very good for heart and artery health. Carnosine is an amino acid found abundantly in red meat, poultry, and seafood; it's also found in our muscles because our bodies produce carnosine from other amino acids. Carnosine is a strong antioxidant that fights free radicals in our bodies, but as we age, our carnosine levels fall. There are many scientific studies that show how important carnosine is for our hearts as well as our muscles, arteries, and brain function. At Ohio University, for example, doctors analyzed carnosine levels in rats (*Comprehensive Biochemistry and Physiology* v 103B, 1992). They discovered that carnosine levels in the heart and skeletal muscles fell over 40 percent as the rats aged, and were 40 percent lower in rats with high blood pressure. Over time, the rats' heart muscles showed a dramatic decline, and the same has basically been found in humans as well. Carnosine helps promote a healthy heart.

DOSAGE: Take 500 to 1,000 mg of carnosine a day, especially if you are a vegetarian, as it is not found in a vegetarian diet.

Di-indolyl Methane

Di-indolyl methane (DIM) is the direct metabolite of indole-3-carbinol or I3C. There are excellent studies on both DIM and I3C that show they lower serum estrogen levels and have anticancer effects. These studies have been published in *Cancer Research*, the *Journal of the National Cancer Association*, *Anticancer Research*, *Annals of the New York Academy of Sciences*, and other major journals. I3C is found in cruciferous vegetables (cabbage, broccoli, Brussels sprouts, and cauliflower), but it is less expensive, and more practical, to take 200 mg a day of DIM rather than 400 mg a day of I3C. DIM is a much better bargain and twice as powerful. High estrogen levels in our bodies cause many problems as we age, but taking DIM is an excellent way to reduce estrogen levels and improve estrogen metabolism. If your levels of free estradiol and estrone test low and normal, you do not need to take this. Maintaining a low-fat diet and exercising can keep estrogen levels low.

DOSAGE: Taking 200 mg of DIM a day can improve your estrogen metabolism.

Fructo-oligosaccharides

Fructo-oligosaccharides (FOS), otherwise known as inulin, works well with glutamine (another important supplement discussed in this chapter) and acidophilus. FOS is an indigestible saccharide that is extracted from various plants (such as chicory) and feeds the good Lacto and Bifido bacteria in our intestines. FOS is called a "prebiotic" and works synergistically with probiotics. The health benefits of FOS have been known for a long time, but it is only recently that the intestinal health benefits have been discovered, and good studies have been published on the subject.

DOSAGE: Take 750 to 1,500 mg of FOS daily, and always remember that 90 percent of our immune system comes from our digestive system.

Glucosamine

Glucosamine is a basic supplement for bone and joint health. Since 95 percent of Americans over the age of sixty-five have some form of arthritis, glucosamine is an important addition to your diet. There is good science behind glucosamine if it is used properly. Glucosamine does not work alone but needs cofactors such as minerals, flax oil, soy isoflavones, and vitamin D; more-over, glucosamine needs hormones such as testosterone, DHEA, estriol, and progesterone.

DOSAGE: Take 500 to 1,000 mg of glucosamine a day. Remember that chondroitin (a supplement derived from animal cartilage that is taken to enhance the elasticity of our own cartilage) is useless despite its popularity—the molecule is too large to pass through the digestive walls and into the blood. Also remember that glucosamine needs cofactors to be effective.

L-glutamine

L-glutamine is an amino acid with many health benefits, espe-cially in strengthening digestive and intestinal function. Several good studies have shown how L-glutamine improves our intes-tinal health, and it works well in concert with acidophilus and FOS. Good digestion is central to good health. Our digestion is generally weak from lifelong dietary abuse, but L-glutamine, along with acidophilus and FOS, improves digestion.

DOSAGE: You should take at least 2,000 mg (four 500 mg tablets) of L-glutamine a day (two tablets in the A.M. and two in the P.M.). You can also buy bulk glutamine powder and take one table-spoon a day; it is tasteless and can be added to your food.

Lipoic Acid

Lipoic acid levels in our bodies fall as we age, and unfortunate-ly, this supplement is not found in our food. There are a lot of excellent scientific studies that suggest that lipoic acid is good for brain metabolism, coronary heart health, and blood sugar metabolism. Insulin resistance and diabetes are epidemics in western society now. One in three American children will grow up diabetic—due mainly to our insane intake of 160 pounds of various sugars every year. Your blood sugar should be 85 mg/dL (milligrams per deciliter) or less, and lipoic acid can help you achieve healthy blood sugar levels. Supplementing you diet with lipoic acid is very important for anyone over the age of forty, or anyone with a blood sugar level over 85 mg/dL.

DOSAGE: You should take 400 mg of regular R,S-lipoic acid a day in order to maintain normal blood sugar levels. Take 400 mg and no less. Do not take R-lipoic acid because it's expensive, and there are no human tests that suggest this substance is actually effective. Nearly all of the clinical studies on lipoic acid have used regular mixed isomer R,S-lipoic acid.

Phosphatidyl Serine

Phosphatidyl serine (PS) is very important for brain function, memory, and preventing Alzheimer's disease and senility. PS is found mostly in our brains and nervous system, and clinical studies on PS have shown that it can help prevent the loss of our mental faculties as we age.

DOSAGE: PS is a very effective supplement, but works best with other brain healthy nutrients, so take 100 mg of PS a day, and use this with ALC and pregnenolone. Only in the last few years has PS become available to us inexpensively from soybeans. Lecithin, or phosphatidylcholine, is also a very good time-proven supplement, especially for heart and artery health. Take 1,200 mg of lecithin a day.

SUPPLEMENTS FOR PERIODIC USE

There are some good exogenous supplements you can take if you like. Exogenous refers to supplements that cannot be found in your body or in your daily food. After about six months, most of the exogenous supplements listed below lose their effect, so only take them for a short period of time.

Aloe Vera

Aloe vera has been known for centuries for its healing power both inside and out. Two 100 mg capsules of a 200:1 aloe vera extract a day, for one year, will help strengthen your digestive system; it can even heal the lining of your stomach and the walls of your intestines. Aloe vera is a time-proven herbal remedy that works well with acidophilus, FOS, and glutamine.

DOSAGE: Take two 100 mg capsules of a 200:1 aloe vera extract a day. Because it is an exogenous supplement, do not take aloe vera for longer than one year.

Curcumin

Curcumin is an extract from the culinary herb turmeric, and it is a powerful anti-inflammatory. A study on prostate cancer at the Comprehensive Cancer Center in New York City showed that curcumin "has the potential to prevent the progression of this cancer . . ." Other articles on curcumin and cancer have been in *Molecular Urology, FEBS Letters, Molecular Medicine*, and other journals.

DOSAGE: Curcumin is a clinically proven anti-inflammatory but should only be used for up to a year because it is exogenous and not found in our bodies or in common foods. Take 500 mg of curcumin daily.

Ellagic Acid

Ellagic acid has shown good anticancer activity in many studies; it can help prevent cancer, stop the growth of tumors, and even kill cancer cells. Because it is commonly found in walnut hulls (as well as in fruits and other nuts), ellagic acid has been known to herbalists for years. Unfortunately, most available brands are overpriced, and their labels are very misleading; they list the amount of extract but not the actual amount of ellagic acid. Find a brand with a label that states 200 mg, or more, of actual ellagic acid. Make sure you don't buy an extract that doesn't state the potency. As research continues, you will hear more about the benefits of ellagic acid in the future.

DOSAGE: Take at least 200 mg of ellagic acid a day. Only take ellagic acid for one year, since it is not found in common food.

Fruit Pectin

Fruit pectin, as part of a total program of diet and supplements, has been shown to help prevent prostate cancer, prostatitis, and BPH. Studies have shown that fruit pectin supplements effectively lower cholesterol and improve digestion. It even has general anticancer properties, so it can prevent and cure various other cancers as well as prostate cancer. Do not waste your money on expensive "modified" pectin. You don't need to modify pectin. Just buy the plain, inexpensive regular kind, like grapefruit or apple pectin. Regular fruit pectin is soluble, bioavailable, and very beneficial in many ways (besides lowering cholesterol levels).

DOSAGE: Take 3 g or more a day, in caplets or as powder (it's tasteless) in fruit juice for up to one year.

Green Tea Extract

Hundreds of published clinical studies on both animals and humans have shown that green tea extract helps alleviate prostate disease. Though most brands contain caffeine, search for a good decaffeinated brand of green tea extract. Green tea contains valuable and powerful antioxidants like polyphenols and cathechins. Yes, this is the same tea you see everywhere, before fermenting changes its color to black. Many inexpensive brands of 95 percent decaffeinated green tea are available. Taking green tea extract supplements is more practical than trying to drink green tea every day.

DOSAGE: Take two 300 mg capsules of 95 percent decaffeinated extract a day. Again, because green tea extract is exogenous, you only need to take this supplement for about a year.

Milk Thistle

Milk thistle has many potential health benefits, particularly for the prostate. Milk thistle is a well-known and time-proven herb because of its powerful active ingredient: silymarin. Studies in many international journals such as *Cancer Letters* and *Cancer Research* have shown that taking milk thistle has very promising effects on our prostate health. This is a very important herb for liver health as well.

DOSAGE: Two capsules a day of a good milk thistle extract will give you about 200 mg of silymarin. After about twelve months you can stop using milk thistle, as all exogenous herbs lose their effect after that time.

Sodium Alginate

Sodium alginate is a seaweed extract that has many proven health benefits. Perhaps the most dramatic benefit of sodium alginate is that it can remove toxic metals from our blood. When sodium alginate binds to radioactive metals (such as mercury, lead, and cadmium) in our blood, these substances are then safely excreted from our bodies through our feces.

DOSAGE: Take 3 g of sodium alginate a day for a year.

Trimethylglycine

Trimethylglycine (TMG), also known as betaine, is an amino acid found in our food. Studies have shown that it has powerful rejuvenating and detoxifying effects on our livers. In fact, TMG is the best liver rejuvenator known to science.

DOSAGE: Take 3 g of TMG a day for up to a year. You can also take 1 g a day permanently to help maintain lower homocysteine levels. (High homocysteine levels are an important diagnostic marker of heart disease.)

SUPPLEMENTS TO AVOID

Over twenty years of research, it has become obvious that most of those "wonder supplements" so heavily promoted on television simply have no scientific evidence behind them. Such products would include resveratrol, ubiquinol, saw palmetto, chondroitin, Pygeum africanum, noni juice, policosanol, deer antler velvet, 5-hydroxytryptamine (5-HTP), homeopathic remedies, bee products (pollen, jelly, propolis, etc.), brewer's yeast, dimethylaminoethanol (DMAE), arginine, hoodia cactus, artemisia (wormwood), shark cartilage, modified (not regular) citrus pectin, Tongkat ali, bilberry, pomegranate products, cetyl myristoleate (CMO), colloidal minerals, coral calcium, salba, PC-SPES, colostrum, chorella, nattokinase, all HGH secretagogues, spirulina, oral chelation, hyaluronic acid, mangosteen products, AHCC, MGN-3, Tribulus terrestis, acai berries, goji berries, astaxanthin, "greens," colon cleansers, Cat's claw (uña de gato), maca root, chrysin, whey protein, suma, muira puama, red rice yeast, oral S.O.D., CLA, Gymnema sylvestre, sexual rejuvenation formulas, and MSM among others.

Even lycopene has no good published science behind it. Actual blood serum studies of lycopene prove that there is no correlation *at all* between lycopene levels and prostate health (the *Journal of the National Cancer Institute* v 82, 1990 and *Cancer Epidemiology Biomarkers Preview* v 6, 1997). At Johns Hopkins University (*Prostate* v 47, 2001), the blood of 25,802 men was analyzed for nutrients and matched with their medical records. *No relation was found with lycopene content.* At the Cancer Research Center in Honolulu (*Igaku No Ayumi* v 103, 1977), the blood of 6,850 men was analyzed for nutrients, and no relation with lycopene levels was found. In fact, tomatoes must be cooked in oil in order for their lycopene to be absorbable. It is clear that actual blood studies on men show no relation at all between serum lycopene levels and prostate health.

AN OVERVIEW OF IMPORTANT DAILY SUPPLEMENTS

The table on page 37 lists the most important supplements you should take on a permanent basis in order to improve the health of your prostate and your health in general. Beside the name of each supplement, you'll find the optimal daily intake, which is not necessarily the same as the reference daily intake (RDI) established by the Food and Drug Administration (FDA). Note, for example, that the RDI for vitamin E is only 30 IU, but the *optimal* daily intake is 200 IU. Vitamin E is very important for prostate health, but most of us don't get enough vitamin E through our normal diets.

TABLE 3.1. PERMANENT DAILY SUPPLEMENTS		
Supplements	Optimal Daily Intake	Considerations
VITAMINS		
Vitamin B_1 (Thiamine)	1.5 mg	
Vitamin B_2 (Riboflavin)	1.75 mg	
Vitamin B_3 (Niacin)	20 mg	
Vitamin B_6	2 mg	
Vitamin B_{12}	2 mg	
Vitamin C	60 mg	Do not take more than 250 mg in one day.
Vitamin D	800 IU	If you are sick or elderly, take up to 1,200 IU a day.
Vitamin E	200 IU of mixed natural tocopherols	Or take 400 IU every other day.
Vitamin K	80 mcg	
Biotin	300 mcg	
Folate (Folic Acid)	400 mcg	
Pantothenic Acid	10 mg	
MINERALS		
Boron	3 mg	
Calcium	250 mg	Some suggest taking 1,000 mg of calcium a day, but only dairy intake will give you this much calcium, and it is better to avoid eating dairy.
Cesium	100 mcg	

TABLE 3.1. Continued		
Supplements	**Optimal Daily Intake**	**Considerations**
MINERALS		
Chromium	120 mcg	
Cobalt	100 mcg	
Copper	2 mg	
Gallium	100 mcg	
Germanium	100 mcg	
Iodine	150 mcg	
Iron	10 mg (men) 18 mg (women)	
Magnesium	400 mg	
Manganese	2 mg	
Molybdenum	75 mcg	
Nickel	100 mcg	
Selenium	70 mcg	
Silicon	10 mg	
Strontium	1 mg	
Tin	100 mcg	
Vanadium	1 mg	
Zinc	15 mg	
OTHER NUTRIENTS		
Acidophilus	6 billion live multi-strain organism capsules	Buy and keep refrigerated. Take once or twice daily.
Acetyl-L-carnitine	500 to 1,000 mg	
Beta-carotene	10,000 IU	
Beta Glucan	200 mg or more	
Beta-sitosterol Complex	300 to 600 mg	

TABLE 3.1. Continued		
Supplements	**Optimal Daily Intake**	**Considerations**
OTHER NUTRIENTS		
Coenzyme Q_{10}	100 mg	If you are ill, take 200 mg daily for one year. Take with food, or flax oil as Coenzyme Q_{10} is oil-soluble.
Di-indolyl Methane (DIM)	200 mg	Take with food, or flax oil as DIM is oil-soluble.
Flaxseed Oil	1,000 to 2,000 mg	Buy and keep refrigerated. Take once or twice daily.
Fructo-oligosaccharides (FOS)	750 to 1,500 mg	
Glucosamine	500 to 1,000 mg	
L-glutamine	2,000 mg	Take two 500 mg tablets in the A.M. and two in the P.M.
Lipoic Acid	400 mg	
N-acetyl Cysteine (Glutathione)	600 mg	
Phosphatidyl Serine (PS)	100 mg	
Quercetin	100 mg	
Soy Isoflavones	40 mg of daidzein and genistein	If you drink soy milk.

CONCLUSION

There are forty-nine permanent supplements recommended in this chapter for men over forty. These are the very same supplements recommended for women, by the way. You should take these supplements in addition to any hormones you need. Use as many supplements listed in Table 3.1 as you possibly can, as they have many overall health benefits. Poor health in general contributes to your prostate condition. Don't choose surgery, radiation, or dangerous prescription drugs because you may end up wearing diapers, losing your sexual ability, or dying a tortuous, premature death. An ounce of prevention is worth ten pounds of cure. These natural, proven products will help both prevent and cure your health problems.

4. The Minerals You Need

S tudies have shown us how important minerals are to prostate metabolism and to health in general. Good mineral nutrition helps us live longer, healthier lives. Though zinc, selenium, and chromium have gotten the most attention, many minerals are vital to our nutrition. Every disease or medical condition is due in part to mineral deficiency. We are all mineral deficient, no matter how well we eat or where we live. We need all the known minerals for human nutrition, not just some of them. Minerals, like hormones, work together as a team. There are at least twenty-four known elements needed for human nutrition. Of those twenty-four, we get enough phosphorous, potassium, sodium, and sulfur in our food, so we do not need to supplement these minerals. The best, most expensive mineral supplements available only have about ten different elements. Few supplements in the world provide all twenty of the minerals we need in the necessary servings, but just google "mineral supplements" to find one that does. A detailed list of these twenty minerals, along with the recommended dosage of each, follows.

BORON

Boron is probably the most deficient mineral in your diet. Americans probably only ingest 1 mg of boron a day, but actually need three times this amount. You would think all vitamin and mineral supplements would contain a mere 3 mg of this inexpensive and vital element, but many do not. This is just another case of megacorporations and manufacturers that have huge advertising budgets but no research departments. It wasn't until 1990 that boron was even considered an essential part of your diet! The research is overwhelming here. Our soils and food are very boron deficient. Boron deficiency is all too common, so be sure to buy a supplement with enough boron.

DOSAGE: There is no official RDI for boron, but 3 mg is commonly agreed to be the suggested daily intake. Citrates or common boric acid are excellent sources of boron.

CALCIUM

Calcium, in any significant quantity, is only found in dairy foods. You should not eat dairy foods. The RDI of 1,000 mg is completely scientifically unfounded. Asians, for example, generally only take in about 250 mg of calcium a day, and they tend to have fewer bone and joint problems than we Americans do.

DOSAGE: Take 250 mg of calcium a day. Be sure to take flax oil, minerals, and vitamin D as well because calcium needs cofactors in order for it to be absorbed.

CESIUM

Cesium is an important ultra-trace mineral, so you only need 100 mcg a day; do not take more than this. Human blood, common food, and soil studies have proven how vital cesium is for our health, and yet you will never find it in mineral supplements. Internationally published studies have also shown the importance of cesium in our soil, our food, and our blood. Cesium is vital for human health, and soon science must admit this fact and set an RDI for cesium.

DOSAGE: Because cesium is an ultra-trace mineral, you only need to take 100 mcg a day. Regular salts, especially chloride, can provide you with enough cesium.

CHROMIUM

Only recently has chromium been given an RDI of 120 mcg. Chromium is often deficient in our diet because we tend to eat refined grains instead of whole grains. Science has proven that chromium is critical for proper prostate metabolism, and chromium deficiency is one of the reasons prostate disease is such an epidemic.

DOSAGE: The RDI for chromium is 120 mcg. Never take more than 400 mcg a day, and do not listen to advertisements that claim their form of chromium is the "only effective one." Regular chelates (nonmetal ions that bond to a metal ion for better absorbability) are the best source of chromium, so simply look for a bottle labeled "chromium chelate."

COBALT

Even though it is the basic building block for vitamin B_{12}, cobalt is never found in mineral supplements. Food and blood studies have proven the importance of cobalt for our health. Our bodies are supposed to synthesize our own vitamin B_{12}, but that process cannot occur without cobalt in our blood. We probably only take in about 25 mcg (or less) of cobalt a day, but that is usually enough; this may not sound like much, but our bodies only need to make about 3 mcg of B_{12} a day. Taking vitamin B_{12} orally just doesn't work, so you must take 1 mg of methylcobalamin daily. Sufficient amounts of vitamin B_{12} are just not found in foods, and B_{12} is ineffective when taken orally. To help insure the production of 3 mcg of vitamin B_{12}, it is actually better to take 100 mcg of cobalt a day. Cobalt is very important.

DOSAGE: In order to insure that your body can produce at least 3 mcg of vitamin B_{12} a day, you should take 100 mcg of cobalt daily.

COPPER

Copper has a low RDI of only 2 mg. Still, Americans probably only consume about half this amount. Whole grains and beans are the best source of copper, but most of us don't eat enough of these foods. Your body only contains about 150 mg of this vital element. That's all. Taking 2 mg of copper a day is good health insurance, but keep in mind that while some people are copper deficient, people with hypertension often have excessive levels of copper. It would take about 15 mg of copper a day for it to become toxic, however, and that is very unlikely.

DOSAGE: Take 2 mg of copper a day. Copper citrates, oxides, and gluconates are all very absorbable.

GALLIUM

Gallium is an ultra-trace element, and gallium nitrate is a good supplement to use. Unfortunately, gallium is rarely found in mineral supplements, and it has been very ignored by science. The few studies we have on gallium are very positive, especially as related to bone metabolism. Gallium is a very overlooked and ignored element.

DOSAGE: Take 100 mcg of gallium a day.

GERMANIUM

Germanium is a very important ultra-trace element, but you will not find it in most mineral supplements. Clinical human blood studies have proven that germanium is vital to our health, but our food, and the soil our food is grown in, is germanium deficient. Germanium sesquioxide and chelates are safe, but germanium dioxide is not, so be careful when selecting the germanium supplement that's right for you.

DOSAGE: You only need about 100 mcg a day of ultra-trace elements like germanium. Do not take more than 100 mcg of germanium a day.

IODINE

Iodine is one of two nonmetallic elements you need to supplement (the other nonmetallic element you need is silicon), and it is very important to your health. Iodine plays a crucial role in balancing your thyroid metabolism. There are only about 30 mg of iodine in your body, and three-fourths of this is in your thyroid gland. Note that there is no reason to use iodized salt; we use too much salt in our diets already, so this is not the best way to get iodine. Surprisingly, regularly eating sea vegetables like kelp, nori, and hijiki (as many Asians do) is not a good idea either. All seaweeds contain extreme amounts of iodine, and overdoses of any mineral can unbalance your metabolism. It's important to note, however, that iodine supplements will *not* correct thyroid problems like hyperthyroidism and hypothyroidism—caused by low levels of the hormones triiodothyronine (T_3) or thyroxine (T_4).

DOSAGE: The RDI of iodine is 150 mcg.

IRON

Iron is the "heme" in hemoglobin, and it's the basic mineral in our blood. Iron deficiency is as common as ever, despite our excessive consumption of red meat. This irony can only be explained by an inability to absorb the iron we need. Iron is rarely found in high levels, and this is due to an excretion problem and not excessive intake. Rather, high blood levels of iron are not caused by consuming too much iron; they are caused by a metabolic problem in which excess iron is retained rather than excreted. If you want to cure your prostate disease, you should stop eating red meat; and if you stop eating red meat, you won't have to worry about an overconsumption of iron.

DOSAGE: Find a good supplement that contains the female RDI of 18 mg or the male RDI of 10 mg. Common sulfates, fumarates, and gluconates make good iron supplements.

MAGNESIUM

Magnesium is generally deficient in western diets because we consume too many refined foods. Whole grains contain plenty of magnesium, but Americans eat a mere 1 percent whole grains—we should be eating at least 30 percent or more! Many illnesses have been correlated to low levels of magnesium in the blood.

DOSAGE: The RDI of magnesium is 400 mg.

MANGANESE

Manganese is a very important mineral for our health, and yet the RDI was only recently established at 2 mg. Whole grains, along with beans and legumes, nuts, and some vegetables, are the major source of manganese, but eating refined foods takes much of the manganese out of our diets. There is an abundance of research about the benefits of manganese for our health. For example, our bodies need manganese for fat metabolism, growth factors, reproduction, muscle coordination, and brain function. Manganese deficiency can result in bone disease, carpal-tunnel syndrome, infertility, and menopausal problems. On the other hand, recent research has shown that manganese supplementation can improve the health of arthritis and osteoporosis patients.

DOSAGE: A 2 mg daily supplement of manganese is good health insurance since we only have around 20 mg of manganese in our bodies. Whole grains, beans, and leafy green vegetables are the best sources of manganese, but sulfates and oxides are effective manganese supplements.

MOLYBDENUM

Molybdenum is safe and nontoxic, even though it is a heavy metal. The research on molybdenum has been more concerned with soils and plants, rather than with animals and humans.

Farmers and gardeners, for instance, commonly use molybdenum in their fertilizer and animal feed. Unfortunately, there has been very little research on the relationship between molybdenum deficiency and various diseases and conditions. However, molybdenum is recognized as an important element for bone and joint health as well as blood sugar metabolism. Anticancer and antitumor properties have been attributed to molybdenum as well.

DOSAGE: Molybdenum has an RDI of 75 mcg. Common salts are good sources of molybdenum, but you will also find this mineral in all your supplement formulas.

NICKEL

Nickel is an ultra-trace element that is often ignored, but 100 mcg a day is all you need. Blood analysis of animals and humans has shown us that nickel is an essential element for our health, but there has been little research on the specific benefits of nickel, or the problems caused by nickel deficiency. The research on nickel has been mostly about mineral deficiencies in our soil and how such deficiencies affect the growth of our crops. Little research has been done on how nickel deficiencies in the food we grow affect our own nutrition, but the few studies we have in this area have shown us some very promising things about nickel. For instance, Chinese children with very high IQs had higher levels of serum nickel than children with average IQs. Nickel also plays an important role in fertility; women with low levels of nickel are more likely to experience infertility or hypertension during pregnancy. People tend to forget about nickel, but it is clearly a very important mineral.

DOSAGE: Supplement your diet with 100 mcg of nickel a day. You won't see nickel in the mineral supplements on the market, but regular salts, such as chlorides and sulfates, are good sources of nickel.

SELENIUM

Selenium has been ignored by nutritionists for decades, but finally the Food and Drug Administration (FDA) has given this essential mineral an official RDI of 70 mcg. Studies show that people with low levels of selenium in their blood are more likely to suffer from cancer, coronary heart disease, and diabetes. Our soils, as well as the heavily refined foods we eat, are very deficient in selenium. Whole grains are the very best source of selenium, and selenium chelates are the most absorbable form of selenium supplement.

DOSAGE: Be sure to take your selenium supplement with 200 IU of vitamin E because selenium and vitamin E work synergistically. Do not exceed a daily intake of more than 200 mcg of selenium, as it is a heavy metal and will accumulate in your body.

SILICON

Sometimes referred to as the "orphan mineral," silicon is another ignored element that is almost never found in mineral supplements. Silicon is the only other nonmetallic elements we need besides iodine, but the lack of silicon supplements just provides more proof that megacorporations have no research departments, only advertising budgets. Silica levels in our foods vary so greatly that it is all but impossible to determine which foods are good sources of silicon; that said, onions, beets, kale, brown rice, and oats are all fine sources of silicon. Unfortunately, there aren't enough studies on the importance of silicon in our diets. We do know, however, that silicon is a basic building block for our bones, cartilage, and tendons; the science here is most impressive. We also know that temporarily taking extra silica gel (or silicic acid) has the unique property of absorbing excess aluminum that's in our bodies and helping us excrete it. This phenomenon is especially crucial since excess aluminum is toxic and builds up in the brains of Alzheimer's patients (not to mention the fact that Americans tend to have high levels of aluminum in our blood). Silicon has many important health benefits, but there need be many more scientific studies on this vital mineral.

DOSAGE: There is no RDI set for silicon, but 10 mg a day is a safe and effective dose. Plain silica gel is a good, inexpensive source of silicon.

STRONTIUM

Strontium is another very important trace element with very good science behind it. You will not find strontium in mineral supplements, but 1,000 mcg a day is a good dose. Like silicon, bone and joint health depend on strontium as a building block, and it's also necessary for calcium absorption. No RDI has been set, but science finally recognizes strontium as an essential part of our nutrition.

DOSAGE: Look for a supplement that has 1,000 mcg—strontium chelates and asparates are good choices—and be careful not to confuse these with the radioactive form: strontium-90.

TIN

Another important ultra-trace element, and one that is often ignored, is tin. Common food and soil studies have proven that tin is an essential element, but most of the research on tin has been concerned with its toxicity (from industrial pollution), instead of with its health benefits. Unfortunately, the FDA irrationally limits the RDI of tin to 30 mcg, and it's difficult to find tin in mineral supplements. Human studies have shown that low blood tin levels are associated with various illnesses, but more research needs to be done on this subject.

DOSAGE: Taking 100 mcg of tin a day is a healthy dose, and regular salts, such as chlorides and sulfates, are good sources of tin and are easily absorbed by our bodies.

VANADIUM

Vanadium also has been ignored by nutritionists until very recently. There is still no RDI for vanadium because it is not considered an essential element. Vanadium has been proven a critical mineral for our health in general, and whole grains and seafood are excellent sources of vanadium, but unfortunately, due to our high intake of refined foods, vanadium deficiency is all too common. There is now very good science on the importance of vanadium. For example, vanadium is extremely important in blood sugar metabolism and diabetes prevention, but it also plays a key role in bone, tooth, and cartilage repair and maintenance. Furthermore, vanadium even has anticancer and antitumor properties.

DOSAGE: Taking 1 mg of vanadium a day is good, but almost no supplements contain this vital mineral. Do not take more than 1–2 mg a day, as vanadium is toxic at 10 mg. Chelates and sulfates are the best vanadium supplements.

ZINC

Zinc levels are generally low in men with prostate disease. Most people do not get the 15 mg RDI they need from the foods they eat. Zinc is found in whole grains, beans, nuts, and meats, but whole grains and beans are the best sources. Zinc deficiency is particularly a problem for the poor, the young and the elderly, and alcoholics. There are about 2.5 g of zinc in the human body, half of which is in the muscles. Zinc is necessary for the synthesis of RNA and DNA, growth and development, reproduction, immunity, and many other bodily processes.

DOSAGE: The RDI for zinc is 15 mg. The usual citrates, oxides, and sulfates all work well as supplements. Even though zinc has a low toxicity level, you should never take more than 50 mg of zinc a day.

CONCLUSION

In the future, it is very possible that we may need other ultra-trace elements such as barium, europium, rubidium, neodymium, praseodymium, thulium, lithium, tungsten, samarium, lanthanum, and yttrium. It is very difficult to determine the effects of these elements since they are needed in such tiny microgram amounts. What is painfully clear is that the mineral supplements on the market are woefully inadequate. It may be challenging to find the right supplements for you, but your health is worth it, and now you know how to choose the safest and most effective mineral supplements. Still, it is always worth remembering how dangerous it can be to take supplements when you don't really understand the ingredients. So always read the label! Supplementing your diet with these vital minerals will set you on your way to a disease-free life.

5. Beta-Sitosterol and Prostate Health

The most proven effective nutritional supplement for prostate health is a common plant alcohol called beta-sitosterol. Beta-sitosterol is found in literally all of the vegetables you eat, and it is the most prominent plant sterol in nature. Actually, beta-sitosterol is really a combination of several sterols, including campesterol, stigmasterol, and brassicasterol. So we really mean mixed sterols when we refer to beta-sitosterol. It is estimated that Americans consume about 300 mg of these mixed plant sterols a day (and those of us who are vegetarians consume about twice that much).

THE TRUTH ABOUT BETA-SITOSTEROL SUPPLEMENTS

Traditionally, herbs such as saw palmetto, *Pygeum africanum*, nettles, and star grass have been used to treat prostate problems. The trouble with using these herbs is that they contain only a tiny amount (one part per three thousand) of the beta-sitosterol complex. A typical analysis of saw palmetto, for example, shows that it contains a variety of fatty acids (capric, eicosenoic, lauric, myristic, palmitic, and others) but only minute (and therefore biologically insignificant) traces of sterols and other plant chemicals. These herbal formulas just do not contain any effective amounts of the active ingredients. You would have to eat a pound of saw palmetto berries in order to obtain a basic dose of 300 mg of beta-sitosterol. Even if you take "10x" extracts of these herbs (with ten times the normal amount of beta-sitosterol), you would still have to eat about 200 capsules, each containing 500 mg, in order to get 300 mg of beta-sitosterol! Analyses published in *Biochemistry, Gazzetta Chimica Italia*, the *Journal of High Resolution Chromatography, the Journal of Pharmacy Science*, and the *Indian Journal of Chemistry* have shown that sterols make up less than 1 percent of these herbs. It is obvious that saw palmetto and other such herbs are ineffective, despite their continual promotion by the so-called natural health industry. Even when the product label reads "85 percent fatty acids and sterols," it usually means "nearly all fatty acids and almost no sterols." Choosing the best beta-sitosterol supplement can be tricky, especially with so many ineffective products on the market, so always read the product label carefully before you try a new supplement.

But what about the herbal extracts sold by prescription in Europe? These extracts are standardized by law according to beta-sitosterol content (regardless of its source), and the beta-sitosterol content is prominently and clearly stated on the label. Whether you buy Permixon in France; Harzol, Tadenan, or Azuprostat in Germany; or Prostaserene in Belgium, these products are all sold according to how much actual beta-sitosterol content they have. Though very expensive, these products are fairly weak. A bottle of sixty tablets of Permixon, for example, containing 30 mg of sterols per tablet, will cost about $50 U.S. You would have to take ten tablets a day to get any benefit, which would cost you about $250 U.S. a month.

After you thoroughly research saw palmetto and *Pygeum africanum*, it is obvious that such herbs are very uneconomical sources of beta-sitosterol; and yet, soybeans, sugarcane pulp, and pine oil (or tall oil from the Swedish "tallolja") are all excellent, natural, and inexpensive sources of beta-sitosterol. Many cane-sugar processors now extract the valuable chemicals from the pulp after the sugar is pressed out. Still, only a few companies sell actual beta-sitosterol supplements containing 300 mg or more. Unfortunately, most popular brands of beta-sitosterol contain insufficient amounts. Find a beta-sitosterol supplement with at least 300 mg of sterols per capsule.

PROSTATE HEALTH BENEFITS OF BETA-SITOSTEROL

There have been dozens of classic double-blind studies on men regarding the effects of beta-sitosterol on BPH or enlarged prostate. We'll discuss a few of these to give you some examples of the first-rate research that has been done around the world at leading hospitals and clinics.

At Ruhr University Bochum in Herne, Germany (*The Lancet* v 345, 1995), Dr. Berges and his associates studied the effects of pure beta-sitosterol on 200 men over the course of a year. Half of the men received beta-sitosterol while the other half received a placebo (in the form of inert capsules). Dr. Berges and his colleagues concluded, "Significant improvement in symptoms and urinary flow parameters show the effectiveness of beta-sitosterol in the treatment of BPH." While this is one of the most important and well-done experiments on prostate health ever published, there are many other noteworthy studies on this subject.

At the Institute of Clinical Medicine at the University of Rome (*European Urology* v 21, 1992), Dr. Di Silverio and his colleagues studied thirty-five men with BPH for three months, giving half of them beta-sitosterol and half of them a placebo. They concluded, "On the basis of these considerations, monotherapy with a special S. repens extract [a clinical high-potency beta-sitosterol extract from *Serenoa repens*, or saw palmetto] may be more favorably accepted, on account of similar clinical results, when compared to the combination therapy cyproterone acetate plus tamoxifen."

A few years later, doctors Wilt and MacDonald at the University of Rome (the *British Journal of Urology* v 83, 1999) gave

Permixon to BPH patients with an average age of sixty-eight. Over a ninety-day period, the addition of Permixon to their diets caused a 50 percent drop in the patients' prostate gland dihydrotestosterone (DHT) levels, and a 72 percent boost in their testosterone levels. This study provides further proof that testosterone is necessary for healthy prostate metabolism, contrary to what many medical doctors believe. (For some reason, many doctors feel testosterone is somehow "bad" for prostate health, even though the clinical research proves that high testosterone levels are correlated with healthy prostates while low levels of testosterone cause prostate disease. Doctors usually give prostate cancer patients hormone treatments that deprive them of testosterone; instead, they should be raising their patients' testosterone levels because 95 percent of men over the age of fifty already suffer from low testosterone.) It is not the serum level of DHT that is critical, but how much DHT binds to the prostate itself. When men don't have enough testosterone to bind to the testosterone receptors on their prostate glands, DHT can bind to those receptors instead. In other words, lowering DHT levels will not actually help improve your prostate health, but raising your testosterone levels will prevent DHT from binding incorrectly to the prostate gland; moreover, beta-sitosterol can also prevent DHT from binding to testosterone receptors. In the same journal, doctors at the Veterans Administration in Minneapolis delivered an extensive review of the research on beta-sitosterol. Going back over thirty years and including thirty-two references, they concluded that beta-sitosterol has "the greatest efficacy amongst phytotherapeutical substances." Furthermore, they found, "Beta-sitosterol improves urological symptoms and flow measures." Since it condenses many studies into one comprehensive presentation, a review like this is very valuable to the field of prostate research.

At the Hospital Ambroise in Paris (the *British Journal of Clinical Pharmacology* v 18, 1984), Dr. Champault and two of his colleagues carried out a classic double-blind study on 110 men, half of whom received a placebo. They concluded, "Thus, as predicted by pharmacological and biochemical studies, PA109 [four tablets of Permixon daily] would appear to be a useful therapeutic tool in the treatment of BPH." Of course, Dr. Champault should have used more beta-sitosterol than that, and if he had, he might have seen even better results.

At the Klinische Endokrinologie in Freiburg, Germany (*Klinische Endokrinologie* v 98, 1980), Dr. Zahradnik and his colleagues demonstrated that beta-sitosterol taken from star grass (and sold as the prescription extract Harzol) lowered prostaglandin levels. It has been shown that high prostaglandin levels support tumor growth, so in order to have a healthy prostate, it's important to maintain low levels of prostaglandin.

Doctors at the University of Padova in Italy (*Minerva Urologica e Nefrologica* v 37, 1985) studied the effect of a special high-potency beta-sitosterol extract (taken from *Pygeum africanum*) on men with BPH. Dr. Tasca and his associates measured urine flow as well as other parameters in men ranging from ages forty-nine to eighty-one, comparing the beta-sitosterol results to the effects from receiving a placebo. The men who received beta-sitosterol achieved a much improved urine flow, but it's important to note that such high-potency extracts are not available to the general public.

In a similar study, Doctor Bassi and his associates at the University of Padova (*Minerva Urologica e Nefrologica* v 39, 1987) analyzed forty BPH patients and the effect of a special high-potency extract of *Pygeum africanum*. Half the men received the beta-sitosterol supplement while half of them received a placebo. The doctors concluded, "The preliminary results demonstrate a significant improvement of the frequency, urgency, dysuria [difficult, painful urination], and urinary flow in patients treated with the active drug."

At the University of Dresden in Germany (the *British Journal of Urology* v 80, 1997), Doctors Klippel, Hilti, and Schipp studied 177 men with BPH for six months. Half of the men received a placebo, and half received the prescription extract Azuprostat containing 130 mg of beta-sitosterol per capsule. To substantiate their research, the doctors cited thirty-two references and carefully screened all the men, who were tested extensively during the study. Dr. Klippel and his colleagues concluded, "These results show that beta-sitosterol is an effective option in the treatment of BPH."

A nine-week double-blind study of fifty men was conducted at the University of Basel in Switzerland (*Urologe A* v 24, 1985). Dr. Vontobel and his colleagues studied a special extract of nettles containing a high concentration of beta-sitosterol. After completing the study, they stated, "The use of beta-sitosterol from nettles, in the evaluation of the objective parameters showed significant differences; the men who received the supplement improved significantly." Unfortunately, you cannot buy such potent extracts in stores.

At eight different urological clinics in Europe (*Wiener Klinische Wochenschrift* v 102, 1990), a collective study on 263 BPH patients was carried out over a two-month period. The patients were given either Tadenan (a *Pygeum africanum* extract with a standardized amount of beta-sitosterol) or a placebo. This very extensive study was coordinated at different clinics among different doctors who all agreed, "Treatment with the Pygeum africanum extract led to a marked clinical improvement. A comparison of the quantitative parameters showed a significant difference between the Pygeum africanum group and the placebo group, with respect to therapeutic response." It's important to realize, however, that the pygeum extracts you buy in the store are much weaker than the extract used in this study. The doctors involved in this study concluded that beta-sitosterol is the most promising medical therapy for treating prostate disease.

A study on twenty-three patients was done at the Urological Clinic of Krankenhaus in Germany (*Medizinische Klinik* v 77, 1982). Over a two-month period, Dr. Szutrely gave patients with prostate enlargement either Harzol (an herbal extract standardized for beta-sitosterol content) or a placebo. He measured their prostates with ultrasound equipment before and after treatment. At the end of the trial he said, "Within the scope of a controlled double blind study to demonstrate the effect of conservative therapy of benign prostatic hyperplasia with Harzol, ultrasonic examination of the prostate adenoma [a benign tumor, which causes prostate enlargement] was carried out on twenty-three patients before and after therapy, with the trial preparation of a placebo. Within a two-month treatment with Harzol there was a significant change in echo structure of the prostate adenoma. This is interpreted as a reduction in the interstitial formation of oedema [or edema, an excess accumulation of fluid in the prostate that causes swelling]."

A unique review by Dr. Wilt at the Department of Veterans Affairs (the *Journal of the American Medical Association* v 280, 1998) of prostate studies examined eighteen different international trials, involving 2,939 men with BPH, that were conducted over a thirty-one-year period. The participants in these trials were given strong extracts of saw palmetto that had been standardized for beta-sitosterol content. After reviewing all these studies, the Dr. Wilt and researchers announced, "The evidence suggests that Serenoa repens (saw palmetto) extract improves urologic symptoms and flow measures."

Another interesting review was conducted by the Department of Urology at the University of Glasgow in Scotland (the *British Journal of Urology* v 78, 1996). Dr. Buck wrote a twelve-page review of herbal therapies, including Harzol, Tadenan, Permixon, Strogen, and Sabalux (all European prescription herbal extracts standardized for beta-sitosterol content), for the prostate. In the review, Dr. Buck discusses the biological basis of prostate illness and documents his report by citing fifty-nine published international studies. His conclusions of the efficacy of herbal treatment are well founded.

In Belgium, Dr. Braekman performed a study at the University of Brussels (*Current Therapeutic Research* v 55, 1994), using

Prostaserene (an extract standardized for beta-sitosterol content). Over a period of three months, some 505 BPH patients were given a twice-daily dose of Prostaserene. Dr. Braekman's observations led him to conclude, "Traditional parameters for quantifying prostatism, such as the International Prostate Symptom Score, the quality-of-life score, urinary flow rates, residual urinary volume, and prostate size were found to be significantly improved after only 45 days of treatment. After ninety days of treatment, a majority of patients (88 percent) and treating physicians (88 percent) considered the therapy effective."

There is another fine review on the effects of beta-sitosterol and BPH from the University of Connecticut (*Pharmacotherapy* v 22, 2002). Dr. Coleman and his colleagues agreed, "In men with BPH, evidence suggests that the agents improve urologic symptoms and flow measures to a greater extent than placebo and to a similar extent as finasteride. Beta-sitosterols also are efficacious in the treatment of BPH, improving urinary symptoms and flow measures in placebo-controlled clinical trials. Phytosterols improved lower urinary tract symptoms (LUTS) and urinary flow measures in numerous clinical trials." The researchers were also very concerned with measuring patients' quality of life (QOL) and concluded, "Based on the studies reviewed, phytosterols are generally well tolerated and potentially effective in treating symptoms of BPH and improving quality of life." This was defined by the International Prostate Symptom Score (IPSS), which was developed in 1993 and is considered to be the gold standard for urological symptoms.

In May 2000, Dr. Berges and his associates at Ruhr University Bochum in Bochum, Germany published another study on beta-sitosterol (the *British Journal of Urology* v 85, 2000). This time, they wanted to carry out a long-term study in order to prove, beyond any doubt, the lasting effects of beta-sitosterol therapy on prostate enlargement. In a classic double-blind study conducted over an eighteen-month period, they measured many basic indexes (such as the IPSS and urine flow) to show in detail how the men fared. While men given only a placebo grew worse with time, those men given beta-sitosterol improved in all measured ways. Dr. Berges and his colleagues concluded, "The beneficial effects of beta-sitosterol treatment . . . were maintained for eighteen months." Clearly, beta-sitosterol is an effective treatment for BPH, even over long periods of time.

CONCLUSION

These are only a few of the many beta-sitosterol studies that have appeared in major medical journals over the last thirty years. Each study shows that beta-sitosterol is the active ingredient in many herbs, including saw palmetto, *Pygeum africanum*, and star grass. American herbal products, even the most expensive extracts that claim to contain "85 percent fatty acids and sterols," have almost no beta-sitosterol in them. Analytical studies prove there are no significant active ingredients in any of these products. This is never mentioned on the label, proving that almost every over-the-counter natural prostate remedy sold in the United States simply has no value. It can be difficult to find a good supplement, especially since most of the beta-sitosterol products used in the studies above are not readily available in your average vitamin shop, but now you know that beta-sitosterol can help cure your BPH. Studies all over the world, at reputable hospitals and clinics, have all confirmed that beta-sitosterol reduces prostate enlargement in men suffering from BPH. No matter how old you are, no matter how sick, beta-sitosterol can improve your health.

6. Other Benefits of Beta-Sitosterol

Beta-sitosterol is the most important supplement to take for prostate health, but it has many other benefits as a daily supplement. Women, for example, should take beta-sitosterol to protect against breast cancer and other breast conditions. Breast cancer is the female equivalent of prostate cancer with the very same causes and the very same cures. Beta-sitosterol can also be used to help treat a wide range of conditions, including high cholesterol, various cancers, diabetes, ulcers, inflammation, poor blood clotting, poor blood parameters, and others. Sterols have antioxidant, antibacterial, antiviral, antimicrobial, and anti-infective properties as well. Everyone over the age of forty should be taking a supplement of at least 300 mg of mixed sterols a day.

BETA-SITOSTEROL CAN LOWER YOUR CHOLESTEROL

The most important benefit of beta-sitosterol is that it can lower cholesterol and triglyceride levels. Coronary heart disease is the biggest killer worldwide by far. Your cholesterol and triglyceride levels are the two most important diagnostic indicators of your heart and artery health. The scientific studies on cholesterol and plant sterols actually go back fifty years, but the general public (and most medical professionals) remains unaware of this.

At McGill University in Montreal (the *Canadian Journal of Physiology* v 75, 1997), a review of decades of scientific literature on beta-sitosterol was conducted. Researchers concluded that the "addition to diet of phytosterols represents an effective means of improving circulating lipid profiles to reduce risk of coronary heart disease." In another study from McGill University (*Metabolism, Clinical & Experimental* v 47, 1998), patients were given plant sterols for just ten days. This was a strict placebo-controlled study in which the patients otherwise continued their normal diets. Total and LDL cholesterol levels were lowered significantly in just ten days.

Perhaps the best beta-sitosterol review of all is from the University of British Columbia (the *American Journal of Medicine* v 107, 1999). This study included eighty-six clinical references dating back to 1951. Researchers discovered that, "In sixteen recently published human studies that used phytosterols to decrease plasma cholesterol levels in a total of 590 subjects, phytosterol therapy was accompanied by an average 10% decrease in total cholesterol and 13% decrease in LDL cholesterol." Moreover, the reviewers noticed an interesting trend in the clinical studies: The worse the diet, the greater the patients' health would improve, and the better the results!

At Uppsala University in Sweden (the *European Heart Journal* Supp. 1, 1999), volunteers were given mixed plant sterols in conjunction with a low-fat, cholesterol-lowering diet. A low-fat diet greatly enhances the beneficial effects of beta-sitosterol, and in less than a month the men and women lowered their total cholesterol a full 15 percent and their LDL cholesterol an amazing 19 percent! This study shows that drugs are not necessary at all. A combination of plant sterols, a reasonable diet, and not even any exercise produced very dramatic results in less than thirty days.

BETA-SITOSTEROL CAN TREAT AND PREVENT CANCER

People who eat more vegetables, and therefore more plant sterols, have lower rates of every known cancer. At Virginia

Polytech Institute (*Cancer Research* v 34, 1974), doctors found that plant sterols are an important factor in preventing colon cancer. The sterols help balance and improve the intestinal flora. Another study on colon cancer was conducted at the Sloan-Kettering Cancer Institute (the *Journal of Cancer Research* v 103, 1982): Merely feeding rats sterols reduced tumor growth and prevented new tumors from growing. Additionally, at Wayne State University (the *Journal of the National Cancer Institute* v 66, 1982) sterols were shown to help prevent intestinal cancer in rats. And at Nihon University in Japan (*Oncology* v 49, 1991) sterols were shown to inhibit skin cancer in mice when researchers simply applied it to the rats' skin. At the State University of New York at Buffalo (the *International Journal of Molecular Medicine* v 5, 2000), beta-sitosterol was found to inhibit both prostate and breast cancer cells. Another fine review from the University of Buffalo (the *Journal of Nutrition* v 130, 2000) revealed that phytosterols in general can help prevent and treat various cancers. This study was complete with a full forty-three references and was most impressive.

BETA-SITOSTEROL CAN CURE BLOOD SUGAR DISORDERS

Diabetes, hyperglycemia, hyperinsulinemia, and insulin resistance are now epidemics in western countries. One in three American children will now grow up diabetic. High blood sugar levels (i.e., over 100) characterize type 2 diabetes. Phytosterol supplementation should be part of a comprehensive program to prevent and treat all blood sugar and insulin conditions. At Dhaka University in Bangladesh (*Pure & Applied Chemistry* v 66, 1994), scientists discovered that beta-sitosterol had hypoglycemic properties that helped lower blood sugar levels in diabetic rats. A similar study at Shiga University in Japan (*Biochemical Biophysical Research Communications* v 186, 1992) confirmed that beta-sitosterol can lower blood sugar levels in diabetic rats. Furthermore, Drs. Ivora and D'Ocon (*Archives Internationales de Pharmacodynamie et de Therapie* v 296, 1988) found that sterols fed to hyperglycemic rats lowered their blood sugar levels; they concluded, "These results indicate a possible anti-hyperglycemic use for the phytosterols in the prevention and treatment of diabetic and pre-diabetic conditions."

BETA-SITOSTEROL CAN TREAT AND PREVENT STOMACH ULCERS

Stomach ulcers are now very common in America. At West China University (*Huaxi Yike Daxue Xeubao* v 23, 1992) plant sterols exhibited antiulcerative properties in rats. The sterols dramatically improved chronic gastric ulcers. A few years later, in another study at West China University (*Huaxi Yaoxue Zazhi* v 11, 1996), the same antiulcerative properties were demonstrated in experimental laboratory animals. Back in the United States, at the University of Texas (*Digestive Science* v 35, 1990), doctors reduced and eliminated gastric ulceration in rats by simply feeding the animals phytosterols. Of their research, the doctors declared, "The results suggest that the sterols may promote the packing of adjacent unsaturated phospholipids . . . to provide the mucosa with protection against luminal acid."

BETA-SITOSTEROL CAN REDUCE INFLAMMATION

Many illnesses involve chronic inflammation, which is basically a complex biological response of our vascular tissues to harmful stimuli. Inflammation results in redness, heat, swelling, and pain, but plant sterols have shown good anti-inflammatory properties. At the Universidade Federal de Santa Catarina in Brazil (*Planta Medica* v 61, 1995), mice were given sterols and then tested for inflammation markers. The mice "exhibited significant analgesic action" and reduced pain from inflammation. Published in the very same journal (*Planta Medica* v 39, 1980), a study conducted at King George's Medical College in India found "potent anti-inflammatory, and analgesic (pain reducing), and anti-pyretic (fever reducing) properties" for sterols. Rats given the sterols in their food achieved dramatic results, and it was concluded, "Sterols possess highly potent anti-inflammatory and antipyretic actions, suggesting its application to human medicine." Finally, in a study at the University of Naples in Italy (*Bulletin of the Italian Society of Biology* v 65, 1989), researchers stated that plant sterols "exhibit moderate anti-inflammatory properties." Doctors and scientists all over the world agree: Beta-sitosterol reduces inflammation.

BETA-SITOSTEROL CAN PREVENT BLOOD CLOTS

What could be more important that the quality of our blood? Plant sterols have been shown to dramatically improve many common blood parameters. At the Tokyo Institute of Technology (*Tanpakushitsu Kahusan Koso* v 30, 1985), doctors published a review—with no less than eighty-nine references—showing the benefits of beta-sitosterol on various blood parameters. In another comprehensive review at the same institute (*Sogo Rinsho* v 34, 1985) sitosterols were again proven to improve blood parameters. Indeed, a third study at the Tokyo Institute (*Medical Philosophy* v 5, 1986) confirmed the results of the first two reviews. With these extensive studies, researchers were looking for a way to prevent blood diseases such as thrombosis (the formation of blood clots). At the Erfurt Medical Academy in Germany (*Folia Haematology* v 115, 1988), scientists discovered further benefits for blood health by simply feeding sterols to laboratory animals. And at Aga Khan University in Pakistan (*Biochemical Society Transactions* v 21, 1993,) even more benefits for blood health were exhibited, including anti-inflammatory and antiplatelet properties. The best study on the benefits of plant sterols on blood parameters was conducted at the University of Stellenbosch in South Africa (the *International Journal of Immunopharmacology* v 18, 1996). There, real human blood cells were analyzed, and various blood cell parameters were very much improved. What's more, the scientists in Stellenbosch provided forty-two full references along with their findings. This research on plant sterols has very important implications for human health, particularly in the prevention and cure of blood clots. Our blood is literally our life stream.

CONCLUSION

There are many other studies we could quote to show the varied benefits of sterols, but even after looking only at those examples listed above, it is obvious that beta-sitosterol is an extremely important part of your diet. Most people do not eat enough vegetables, so they do not get the sterols they need. Be sure to take 300 to 600 mg a day of mixed sterols to improve not only your prostate health but also your health in general.

7. Curing Prostatitis and Prostate Cancer

Along with BPH, prostatitis and cancer of the prostate are the most common forms of prostate disease. These conditions affect millions of men every year, and unfortunately, most of these men do not receive the proper treatments. Most medical doctors today treat prostate disease with hormone therapy, surgery, or radiation, but the truth is, there is much safer and more effective way to cure your prostate disease. This chapter discusses how to prevent, treat, and ultimately cure prostatitis and prostate cancer.

PROSTATITIS

Prostatitis is the chronic inflammation of the prostate gland. All too common in western countries but rare in rural regions of Asia, prostatitis can be a very painful and debilitating condition. This inflammation is due to low immunity in the reproductive area. Many factors contribute to low immunity, but poor diet is the main cause; in fact, 90 percent of our immunity comes from our digestive system. Americans eat twice as many calories as they need—a full 40 percent fat calories, twice the necessary protein, 160 pounds of various sugars, and only 1 percent whole grains. Other factors contributing to low immunity include hormone imbalance, stress (physical and emotional), lack of exercise, taking prescription drugs, alcohol use, smoking, and regular use of caffeine. When your immunity is impaired, your body cannot cure itself and effectively fight off illnesses. Attacks of prostatitis can be triggered by various factors including anal intercourse (heterosexual or homosexual), urethitis (urinary tract infections), cystitis (bladder infections) or postsurgical complications.

Preventing Prostatitis

How can you strengthen your immunity? With a total program of diet and lifestyle. Nothing less. The main thing is to eat well. Take proven supplements. Balance your basic hormones. Exercise. Fast one day every week. Do not take prescription drugs, except for short-term emergencies. Drink in moderation, or don't drink at all. Don't smoke. Give up caffeine. Specifically, there is a one-year program you can follow to strengthen your digestive system, and therefore strengthen your immune system. Eat two meals a day. Eat only macrobiotic food. Don't eat out, and pack your lunch for work. Take acidophilus and FOS in the morning, and then again in the evening. Buy bulk glutamine and take one tablespoon a day. Take two aloe vera capsules a day. Follow this regimen for a year, and your digestive system will be renewed. You can also rejuvenate your liver by taking 3 g (six capsules) of TMG a day for six months. Your liver is essential to your digestion. Strengthening your immunity is going to take time and patience, but you will get results every month. You are going to have to treat yourself with a total program of diet and lifestyle if you want to cure an inflamed prostate gland and keep it cured. Prostatitis is actually more difficult to cure than outright prostate cancer since it is chronic and due to lowered immunity.

Detecting and Treating the Disease

Most cases of prostatitis are simply the chronic variety with moderate swelling, inflammation, and discomfort. Acute chronic prostatitis is a much more dangerous affair. Men can suffer from chills, fever, pain in the reproductive area, burning urination, and frequent urination. This can easily be diagnosed by finding white blood cells and bacteria in the urine. There are many types of bacteria that cause this, such as E. coli, klebsiella, and proteus. The usual medical treatment is powerful bactericidal antibiotics, such as doxycycline, that kill the bacteria outright. (Bacteriostatis antibiotics like tetracycline merely slow down bacterial growth.) The bacteria are not causing the problem at all. The bacteria can only grow because of an impaired immune system that would normally control their development. Such treatments, of course, are purely symptomatic, and do nothing to deal with the cause of the bacterial assault. In fact, these antibiotics harm the digestive system and kill off the good digestive bacteria in our stomach and intestines, so the patient ends up in worse shape than ever. Yet such antibiotic therapy often is repeated regularly. Often patients who receive no medical treatment at all recover just as quickly as those who do. Doctors have also resorted to prescribing alpha-blockers, anti-inflammatories, physiotherapy, and even surgery, all to no avail.

There is also a condition called nonbacterial prostatitis in which no invading bacteria can be determined in the urine. The symptoms here are blood in semen, blood in urine, pain in the genital area, frequent urination, burning urination, weak urine stream, pain with ejaculation, and pain during bowel movements. Taking antibiotics in such cases is useless. Doctors can do nothing here but take your money and worsen your health with toxic prescription drugs.

Facing the Facts

Prostatitis, or any slight infection of the prostate, can falsely raise your prostate-specific antigen (PSA) levels. This often leads to damaging and very unnecessary biopsies. This is just further proof the PSA is not an accurate diagnostic tool at all and should be abandoned. More and more researchers are admitting the PSA is inaccurate, misleading, and should be dropped. The inventor of this test said it is a waste of time and money. Biopsies are never called for, and only about one quarter of men who get them have cancer.

Unfortunately, there is very, very little scientific research on the natural treatment of prostatitis. The only research available is primarily concerned with using dangerous prescription drugs to cover up the symptoms of disease. What little research there is on natural cures, however, is all very promising. At the Institute for Male Urology in California (*Urology* v 54, 1999) a double-blind study was done. Men with prostatitis were given 500 mg of quercetin twice a day for a month, though half of them were really given a placebo. The men who received the quercetin improved their health by 25 percent, without any change to diet or lifestyle. The men who received the placebo did not experience any improvement in their disease. A similar study using quercetin was conducted at the University of California at Los Angeles Harbor Medical Center (the *Journal of the American Nutraceutical Association* v 2, 1999), and this clinical trial also produced positive results. Just taking a natural antioxidant like quercetin helps cure prostatitis. Imagine the results you could have if you took quercetin and other supplements in conjunction with a total program of diet and lifestyle.

PROSTATE CANCER

Prostate cancer is *the* leading cancer for American men, and the second leading cause of cancer mortality. Most men will eventually have cancer cells in their prostate, unless they change their diet and lifestyle. Prostate cancer is clearly caused by poor diet and lifestyle—this is the mirror image of breast cancer in women, with the same causes and natural cures. Saturated animal fat is the main cause of prostate (and breast) cancer, plain and simple. Just look at Figure 7.1, Incidence and Mortality of Prostate Cancer in Developed and Undeveloped Regions. There is a twenty-five times difference between the lowest and the highest rates, and this is due to diet and lifestyle.

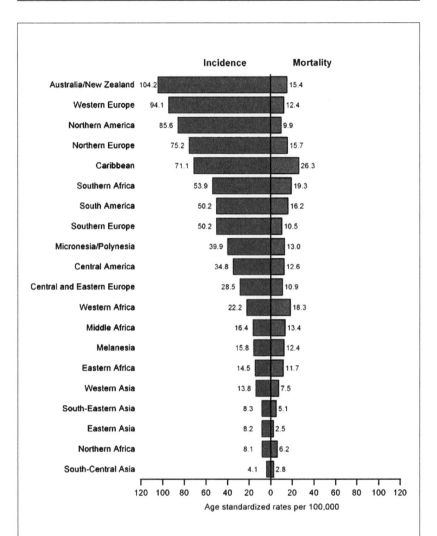

FIGURE 7.1. Incidence and Mortality of Prostate Cancer in Developed and Undeveloped Regions. This figure compares the incidence of prostate cancer across twenty different regions, including both developed and undeveloped parts of the world. Note that North America has one of the highest rates of prostate cancer. Those in less industrialized regions of the world (who consume less fatty and highly-processed foods) are much less likely to develop prostate cancer. Also note the prostate cancer-related mortality rates depicted in this figure; while North America does not have the highest mortality rates, 9.9 out of 100,000 is certainly nothing to be proud of.

Preventing Prostate Cancer

This is a very slow-growing cancer. One in six American men is walking around with cancer cells in his prostate gland. Early detection is not the answer at all; prevention is the answer. Taking meat, poultry, eggs, and dairy foods out of your diet is the answer.

Detecting and Treating the Disease

There are no symptoms in the beginning. The PSA test is not reliable at all—don't even waste your time—the inventor of this test even said it should be dropped. Get a sonogram, an MRI, or even a color Doppler (a advanced kind of ultrasound) to actually see an electronic photograph of your prostate gland. Never, ever get a biopsy for any reason. Biopsies only stimulate cancer growth and are not needed. The symptoms do not show up until the cancer is very advanced. Burning urination, difficult urination, and blood in the urine can be signs of cancer, or signs of mere BPH. In its last stages, cancer can produce symptoms such as fatigue, malaise, weight loss, abdominal pain, back and chest pain, and jaundice.

The prostate cancer industry is about money, money, and more money. The standard treatments are incredibly expensive, yet they merely cover up the symptoms and leave the cause intact. Surgery, radiation, drugs, and chemotherapy leave the patient with no quality of life at all. Diapers and impotence are the usual outcome, and then the poor man will typically die anyway.

Yes, prostate cancer can be cured naturally, without resorting to surgery, radiation, drugs or chemotherapy. Prostate cancer may actually be cured by diet alone. The best book on this subject is *Confessions of a Kamikaze Cowboy*. The author and actor Dirk Benedict *(The A-Team)* got prostate cancer in his thirties, at the height of his career. He decided to go on a macrobiotic diet and stopped eating meat, poultry, eggs, dairy, refined foods, tropical foods, alcohol, coffee, and sugars of any kind. Of course, Dirk did not have the many supplements and hormones we have now.

The doctors wanted to castrate him, which meant he would die anyway, and with a terrible quality of life. Dirk thought about this option, and decided that the whole grain diet, and living another fifty years, sounded better than dying a painful and premature death, with no testicles. He turned his back on the doctors completely and refused all medical treatments. Within seven months Dirk knew he was basically well, and would soon be completely cancer-free. Over thirty years later, Dirk is happy, healthy, youthful, and the father of two handsome sons. This inspiring book, relating his true-life story, is vitally important to read. Other great books on this subject include Anthony Sattarilo's *Recalled By Life* (out of print, but at libraries), Mina Dobic's *My Beautiful Life*, and Elaine Nussbaum's *Recovery From Cancer*.

The most important factor in curing prostate cancer, or any other cancer, is to change your diet and lifestyle. Stop eating eggs, dairy, poultry, meat, and sugars of any kind (even honey and maple syrup). Avoid tropical foods, coffee, hydrogenated oils, preservatives and chemicals, and refined foods. Don't smoke cigarettes, take prescription drugs, or drink alcohol. A diet based on whole grains, beans, most vegetables and some local fruit, soups and salads, and small amounts of seafood (if you don't want to be a vegetarian) is the way to cure yourself. There are various books available on the macrobiotic diet, and there are some fine authors out there who have written books on the natural diet, including Susan Powter, Robert Pritikin, Dean Ornish, and others (as discussed in Chapter 1). Unfortunately, the vast majority of diet books are not good at all—to put it mildly.

As discussed earlier, whole grains such as rice, wheat, barley, and oats are literally the staff of life. They have been the dietary basis of most cultures for thousands of years. Eating well also means eating low-fat, low-calorie foods, and, as stated in Chapter 1, researchers at the Hutchison Cancer Center (*Cancer Epidemiology Biomarkers Preview* v 11, 2002) have shown that low-calorie diets help cure prostate cancer in men.

After you have changed your diet, the second most important thing to do is to take the proven supplements for your general health. Nothing can compensate for not eating well, but the supplements recommended in this book are safe, natural, inexpensive, effective, and proven—in medical journals around the world—to support good prostate health.

Fasting is another powerful treatment for healing cancer. Fasting just one day per week (supper one day to supper the next day, drinking only water) can change your health completely. Fasting is literally *the* most powerful healing method known. Some fine books on fasting have been written by Paul Bragg, Joel Fuhrman, Eve Adamson, Nathaniel Bronner, and Allan Cott. Please remember that true fasting means nothing but water. If you feel you can't fast and go without food, then go on a diet of, say, only brown rice for a period of time. You can also go on a low-calorie, soup-only diet. Soon you will be able to fast one day a week with no problem. People think of fasting as starvation, deprivation, and hunger; actually, hunger pangs generally go away after the second day, and a feeling of lightness, elation, and joy takes over. Besides being a powerful healing method, fasting also develops character and spirituality.

The final step in curing your prostate cancer is hormone balancing. The prostate is strongly hormone-controlled. Saliva testing of hormones is the greatest medical breakthrough in the last decade. Most of the public is still completely unaware of it, as are medical professionals. Doctors rarely test hormone levels, and have little knowledge of how to do this properly. Hormones are very powerful, are not to be used casually, and should not be taken without first testing your levels. Hormone testing will become very mainstream in the near future. Dehydroepiandrosterone (DHEA), testosterone, pregnenolone, progesterone, melatonin, thyroid (T_3 and T_4), human growth hormone (HGH), and cortisol levels are all critical to good prostate health. If you wish to maintain the youthful hormone levels you had in your thirties, you can use a hormone supplement and monitor your levels annually, but we will discuss hormone balancing in greater detail in the next chapters.

Prayer is also effective if you have any religious orientation. It is the sincerity of your prayer that counts. Faith is simply trust in the unknown, and trust can and does move mountains. Prayer works.

Recently, a theory called "complementary medicine," which uses both conventional allopathic (which tends to treat only the symptoms) and natural (which treats only the cause) medicines, has been popularized. But you cannot go north and south at the same time, and you cannot successfully use opposing methods of healing. The best way to get well is to use allopathic medicine only for the effective diagnostic techniques it employs. You then have a choice of completely avoiding radiation, chemotherapy, prescription drugs, and surgery. These medical methods merely disguise your symptoms and ignore the causes of your illness. Use natural treatments to deal with the very cause of your illness. Surgery, radiation, and chemotherapy cannot be reversed. The damage is permanent.

Facing the Facts

Simply dieting and changing your lifestyle may not seem like a very effective treatment plan for prostate cancer, but the fact is, it works. Below are just two accounts—out of dozens—from men who have completely cured themselves of prostate cancer with diet and supplements, and *without* surgery, radiation, or prescriptions drugs.

A classic success story of naturally healing prostate cancer comes from my friend Laddie in Oregon. In his fifties, he found he had prostate cancer, it was verified, and the diagnosis was he would probably be dead within five years, no matter how many medical treatments he underwent. Laddie said he would rather die of cancer than undergo such torture. His wife, Monica, was determined not to be a widow, and looked into the natural healing of cancer. She read up on macrobiotics and immediately put Laddie on a diet of whole grains, beans, most vegetables, local fruits, and some seafood. All his life Laddie had eaten meat, eggs, poultry, dairy, sugar, alcohol, coffee, and refined foods—the usual American diet. He decided it was time to change his diet and lifestyle. Monica made his meals every day, packed his lunch, and made sure he stayed with the diet and didn't deviate.

Laddie bought all the supplements recommended in this book, and took them every day. Taking supplements was the easy part. They were a fraction of the cost of the toxic prescription drugs he would have used otherwise. He took melatonin and pregnenolone, and used transdermal progesterone cream daily. His thyroid was fine, but with saliva testing he discovered that his testosterone and DHEA levels were both low. Laddie went against the advice of his doctor, who believed testosterone is bad for the prostate and increases cancer growth. Laddie raised his low levels of testosterone and DHEA.

Laddie had never gone without food for more than twelve hours in his life, but he started fasting for twenty-four hours, once a week, by skipping breakfast and lunch every Saturday. He also started going on occasional two-day fasts. He knew he was getting well because he FELT better. Healthy people feel good. You could just look at him and see he was getting healthier month-by-month. His friends and relatives felt pity for him, and thought he was in extreme denial. Laddie lost weight, his complexion became clearer, he had more energy, and he simply looked and felt better. His original doctor became very upset as Laddie grew healthier and healthier every month, refusing all traditional medical treatments. He told the doctor he had raised his testosterone levels and was taking four other natural hormones. The doctor became so frustrated that he stopped seeing Laddie and referred him to a colleague!

After less than eight months, Laddie knew in his heart he was well. He had never felt or looked better in his life. Since the PSA is such an unreliable test for diagnosis, he got a sonogram, which showed no more malignancy. His second doctor verified that there was no longer find any evidence of cancer in Laddie's body. He tried to tell Laddie that there must have been a "mistake," and that he never had cancer, but Laddie showed him the original diagnostic results. Today, Laddie is a happy, healthy, and thankful man. He eats well, takes his supplements and hormones, and fasts once a week to celebrate being alive. He expects to live into his nineties.

Bob Young is an eighty-year-old, blind jazz musician who lives in New Jersey, and his is another success story about using natural methods to heal prostate cancer. Bob was diagnosed with prostate cancer fourteen years ago, but he refused the conventional medical treatments. He heard one of my radio shows and finally tracked me down on the phone. Since he couldn't read, I sent him some audiotapes to listen to, and spoke with him over the phone. His aides also read him my books regularly. He changed his diet and quit eating meat, eggs, poultry, and all dairy products. He started eating whole grains and other natural foods. He took all the suggested supplements and tested his basic hormones. Unlike Laddie's medical doctor, Bob's doctor was very supportive of his natural treatment, and helped him test his hormones. It took two years because of his advanced, long-term tumor growth and his age, but Bob finally was diagnosed cancer-free, both by MRI and sonogram. He enjoys his natural food diet, still takes sixteen supplements every day, and keeps his hormones in balance. Bob is looking forward to another good ten years of life, and plays in his jazz band weekly. If an elderly blind man can cure his cancer by changing his lifestyle, then you can, too. Bob is an inspiration to anyone with a serious illness.

There are many other true-life stories of men who cured prostate cancer naturally on my Web site library, which you can find at www.YoungAgain.org/Library.html. Remember, you can cure your prostate cancer in only one year just by changing your diet and lifestyle.

CONCLUSION

The scientists of the world should do a lot more research on natural cures—not only for prostatitis and prostate cancer, but also for BPH. Unfortunately, there is just no profit in studying inexpensive, unpatented, nonprescription supplements and hormones, much less diet and lifestyle. The profits come from studying expensive prescription drugs, so that is where most all of the research is going.

Nevertheless, now that you know how to effectively cure your prostatitis, or your prostate cancer, you can look forward to a longer, happier life. You don't have to be one of those men who suffers through hormone therapy, surgery, or chemotherapy. You can improve your health significantly by simply changing your diet and lifestyle.

8. Your Basic Hormones

The prostate gland is very much influenced by your hormones. It is vital that you have youthful levels of your basic hormones. We are going to discuss progesterone, DHEA, melatonin, pregnenolone, the human growth hormone, T_3 and T_4, insulin, cortisol, and thymus hormones, but there is a complete list of basic hormones on page 82. Note that estrogens and testosterone are covered in later chapters.

PROGESTERONE

Progesterone is thought of as a female hormone, but it actually protects both men and women from excess estrogen. Men need progesterone in their bodies, too, only in smaller quantities than women. The estrogens estradiol and estrone are the feminizing hormones in men, and it is progesterone that is the natural antagonist to them. Excessive estrogen levels in men over fifty cause cancer, breast growth, obesity, and other health problems, but progesterone can help inhibit estrogens.

Nature has given progesterone to both men and women in order to balance and offset the strong effects of estrogen. Men, of course, have naturally lower levels of progesterone than women, so they need less supplementation. Be careful not to confuse real, natural progesterone with progestins (synthetic progesterones) like Provera® that have been shown to cause serious side effects. Progestins do not have the advantages of natural progesterone. Men have specific progesterone receptors on their prostates to which no other hormone can attach, so clearly a healthy prostate requires progesterone; yet, even many urologists and endocrinologists are blind to such well-known scientific facts. This fact was demonstrated over thirty years ago, when doctors at Flinders Medical Center in Australia (the *Journal of Steroid Biochemistry* v 12, 1980) suggested progesterone therapy as a treatment for prostate disease, but no one listened. In the book *Progesterone and Progestins* (Raven Press 1983), the doctors at Service de Medicale in Paris noted that progesterone was vital for proper prostate health. Progesterone protects men from both estrogen dominance and over activity of 5-alpha reductase. *Your prostate needs progesterone to be healthy.*

Now, let's quickly discuss the research that shows progesterone opposes and balances excess estrogen, and is a powerful 5-alpha-reductase inhibitor. This means progesterone helps prevent the conversion of beneficial testosterone into dihydrotestosterone (DHT). High levels of DHT are a major cause of

---

The Basic Hormones in Your Body

This chapter focuses on several hormones that are important to the well-being of your prostate. Below, you'll find a list of all the basic hormones necessary for prostate health.

- Androstenedione
- Cortisol
- Dehydroepiandrosterone (DHEA)
- Estradiol
- Estrone
- Estriol
- Human Growth Hormone (HGH)
- Insulin
- Melatonin
- Pregnenolone
- Progesterone
- Testosterone
- Thyroxine (T_4)
- Triiodothyronine (T_3)

prostate disease, particularly because your prostate will incorrectly accept DHT instead of real testosterone if you have low testosterone levels. We've seen that men over fifty only have about half the testosterone they should; moreover, they also generally have very high levels of both estradiol and estrone.

The very best study on progesterone was conducted almost forty years ago at the Faculty of Medicine in Paris (the *Journal of Clinical Endocrinology and Metabolism* v 38, 1974). Men were given real transdermal progesterone (groundbreaking at the time), which dramatically inhibited the conversion of testosterone into DHT. The researchers suggested progesterone as a standard therapy for men with prostate disease. This is an important and powerful study, but unfortunately modern day urologists have largely ignored it. There are many, many animal and cell studies on the benefits of progesterone for prostate disease, but almost no human studies, and there have not been more studies using transdermal progesterone on real men. Instead, doctors are studying toxic, dangerous, ineffective, and very expensive patentable prescription drugs.

The Center for Drug Research in India performed four different studies that all showed how progesterone shrank enlarged rat prostates and moderated the stimulating effects of estrogen. The main study was published over forty years ago in *Endokrinologie* (v 55, 1970). Just giving progesterone to rats with BPH resulted in significantly reduced prostate volumes—and in only thirty days. This is nothing less than amazing. Well-done animal studies like this are very important precursors to human studies. There are many such studies in the scientific literature, yet no human research is being done anymore on real men.

At Montreal General Hospital (the *Journal of Clinical Endocrinology and Metabolism* v 39, 1974), researchers showed that progesterone strongly inhibited DHT formation in men. "The ability of progesterone to inhibit DHT formation represents one mode of action which may account at least in part for their efficacy in treating BHP." This happened almost forty years ago.

At the Institute of Clinical Chemistry in Germany (*Prostate* v 6, 1985), doctors discovered that progesterone inhibited 5-alpha reductase in human prostates. This is what converts "good" testosterone into "bad" DHT. Researchers at St. George's Hospital in London found the same effect (the *Journal of Endocrinology* v 63, 1974): Progesterone was dramatically effective in inhibiting 5-alpha reductase and the conversion of testosterone into DHT. Similar results were demonstrated at the University of Mainze in Germany (the *Journal of Steroid Biochemistry* v 6, 1975).

DOSAGE: You do not have to test your progesterone levels, and saliva testing does not work well anyways, as progesterone is fat-soluble. Progesterone is poorly absorbed orally. If taken by mouth, it is broken down into unwanted metabolites. Fortunately, progesterone is readily absorbed through the skin into the bloodstream; therefore, transdermal creams are very practical and effective. Find a good brand that contains 800–1000 mg of natural, pharmaceutical grade (standardized for quality assurance by the United States Pharmacopeia, or USP) progesterone per two-ounce jar (400–500 mg per ounce); these specifications should be stated clearly on the label. Apply one-eighth of a teaspoon of the cream directly to your scrotum five days a week. You can also dab it on your inner wrist if you want. Regular application of the cream allows the progesterone to penetrate the skin and reach the prostate receptors. Just one-eighth of a teaspoon provides about 7 mg, of which about 2 mg should be absorbed into your system. Progesterone is completely nontoxic and very safe, especially in these small amounts.

DEHYDROEPIANDROSTERONE

Dehydroepiandrosterone (DHEA) is the second-most important androgen for prostate health after testosterone. DHEA is very important for male sexual and urological health. Men with erectile dysfunction often suffer from low levels of DHEA and need

FIGURE 8.1. DHEA Sulfate Levels Throughout Life. This figure depicts the average man's DHEA sulfate levels throughout his life. Note that levels usually peak around age twenty. And by the time he turns forty, a man's DHEA levels are typically only half what they were at his physical peak.

supplementation. DHEA is called the "life extension hormone" for good reason. Many diseases, including coronary heart disease, show evidence of low levels of DHEA in patients. DHEA levels also fall as we age, as you can see from Figure 8.1, DHEA Sulfate Levels Throughout Life.

In one study, men with prostate cancer had their blood analyzed, which revealed decidedly lower DHEA levels than healthy controls (*Urology Times* v 26, 1998). Similarly, at Johns Hopkins University, researchers compared the DHEA levels of men with prostate cancer to those of healthy men. The prostate cancer patients (*Cancer Epidemiology Biomarkers* v 2, 1993) had 12 percent lower DHEA levels than the healthy men. Other studies have shown that, in general, higher DHEA levels can help prevent prostate disease.

At the University of Vienna (*Prostate* v 44, 2000), men with prostate cancer were compared to healthy controls. The doctors concluded, "These data are confirmed by the present study; it can be concluded that DHEA or DHEA-S serum concentrations represent no risk factor for prostate cancer development." This couldn't be clearer.

At the Urologische Klinik in Budapest (*Magyar Onkologia* v 14, 1970) over forty years ago, doctors studied prostate cancer patients and found that the men had low levels of DHEA. They suggested that such patients be treated with DHEA to normalize their levels.

At the Institute of Endocrinology in Berlin (*Experimental and Clinical Endocrinology & Diabetes* v 99, 1992) doctors found, "DHEA levels in patients with prostate cancer were significantly lower."

At Huddinge University in Sweden (*Prostate* v 13, 1988), doctors performed an in-depth study, involving ten different hormones, of seventy-eight men with prostate cancer. The research showed that men with high, youthful levels of DHEA and DHEA-S had a much better prognostic outlook, especially with regards to whether the cancer spread and metastasized. This excellent study included twenty-two references. Whether the cancer metastasizes is critical to the length and quality of life.

DOSAGE: You can take 25–50 mg of DHEA a day, but there is no established RDI for this hormone yet, so it is better to test your DHEA levels in order to arrive at a dose that's right for you.

MELATONIN

In 1958 melatonin was identified as the pineal gland hormone, but it wasn't until the mid-1990s that it became available as an inexpensive supplement. There has been extensive research done on the prostate health benefits of melatonin, yet we never hear about any of this. The hallmark of this research is the discovery that the prostate actually contains melatonin receptors. Yet many medical doctors, including urologists, are not aware of this fact, and most of the books on prostate health fail to discuss melatonin. Figure 8.2, Melatonin Levels Throughout Life, shows that melatonin peaks around age thirteen and then falls severely until it almost disappears around age sixty.

At the University of Lodz in Poland (*Neuroendocrinology Letters* v 20, 1999) doctors showed that melatonin has beneficial effects on cancer in general. They said, "Melatonin may exert its oncostatic (cancer defeating) effect indirectly, via modulation of the endocrine and immune systems." Other researchers at the University of Lodz (the *International Journal of Thymology* v 4, 1996) came to the same conclusion: Melatonin should be used as a standard means of treating prostate cancer. "Moreover," they stated, "preliminary results of use of melatonin in the treatment of cancer patients suggest possible therapeutic role for melatonin in human malignancy." So why isn't melatonin supplementation used as a standard cancer therapy now?

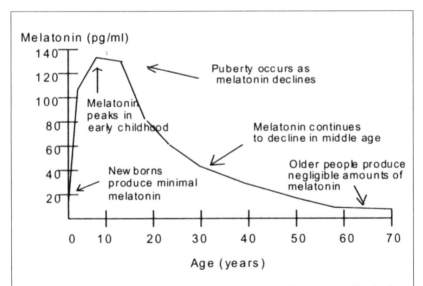

FIGURE 8.2. Melatonin Levels Throughout Life. This figure illustrates how melatonin levels fall as you age. Unfortunately, melantonin levels tend to peak around age thirteen. After that, the amount of melatonin in our bodies falls steadily, and by the time we are sixty, we have almost no melatonin left.

At the San Gerardo Hospital in Milan (*Prostate* v 45, 2000) researchers discovered dramatic benefits after giving melatonin to men with prostate cancer. The doctors reported (the *Journal of Pineal Research* v 2, 1985) that men with BPH and prostate cancer had low melatonin levels, and that melatonin therapy should be used for these conditions. Doctors in China (*Zhongguo Yaolixue Tongbao* v 24, 2008) published a heavily referenced review on the melatonin studies and concluded, "Melatonin is a promising agent for cancer treatment and prevention." Researchers at the University of Hong Kong (the *Journal of Pineal Research* v 43, 2007) also called for, "the use of melatonin in prostate cancer prevention" due to its proven effectiveness.

As a result of all the impressive animal studies, scientists have also conducted human studies on the benefits of melatonin. At the University of Tübingen in Germany (*Clinica Chimica Acta* v 209, 1992), researchers realized that men with both BPH and prostate cancer had low melatonin levels. In a later study at the same university (*Wiener Klinische Wochenschrift* v 109, 1997), doctors observed the same phenomenon in men with prostate cancer. The doctors suggested that using melatonin supplements to treat prostate cancer should be a standard form of therapy. A third study (*7th Colloquium of the European Pineal Society*, 1996) found low levels of melatonin in prostate cancer patients. A fourth study (*International Congressional Series*, 1993) strongly recommended giving melatonin to all men with prostate cancer as standard therapy. Other researchers at the University of Tübingen composed a long review of prostate cancer studies (*Advances in Experimental and Medical Biology* v 467, 1999) that included seventy-one references, all of which consistently showed that breast and prostate cancer patients have low levels of melatonin; again, the reviewers suggested using melatonin supplements as part of standard therapy. The sixth study (*Neuroendocrinology Letters* v 5, 1983) emphasized the "dynamic" effect of melatonin on prostate cancer growth. Men with both BPH and prostate cancer were found to have low melatonin levels.

For years, medical doctors and researchers all over the world have been recommending melatonin supplements as a standard treatment for prostate cancer, but because their research has not been greatly publicized, most people don't know how beneficial melatonin really is.

DOSAGE: Take melatonin supplements only at night, never during the day. Research has shown that taking up to 3 mg a night is a safe and effective dose, but you may not need this much. The media has tried to portray this hormone as a mere sleep aid when, in fact, it is a powerful and proven antiaging, anticancer antioxidant that stimulates the immune system. Melatonin is a very powerful hormone!

PREGNENOLONE

Pregnenolone is the "mother" hormone from which all other sex steroid hormones are derived. It is most important as a brain metabolism regulator as it is largely responsible for memory, learning, and cognition. Pregnenolone might be called the forgotten hormone, as very little research has been done on its role in the endocrine system. Pregnenolone is the most potent memory enhancer known to science, and yet even many endocrinologists are basically unaware of how important it is to measure and supplement pregnenolone, especially in people over the age of forty. Why has there been so little research on such a basic and powerful hormone?

As Figure 8.3 shows, pregnenolone falls precipitously after the age of thirty-five. Saliva testing kits for pregnenolone can be purchased on the Internet, and blood tests can be specially ordered by your doctor. Very little research has been done on pregnenolone and prostate health in the last three decades. Fortunately, at the famous Marie Curie Hospital in Paris (the *Journal of Steroid Biochemistry and Molecular Biology* v 46, 1993) doctors carried out an extensive, unusually sophisticated, and very detailed study on pregnenolone. They measured the levels

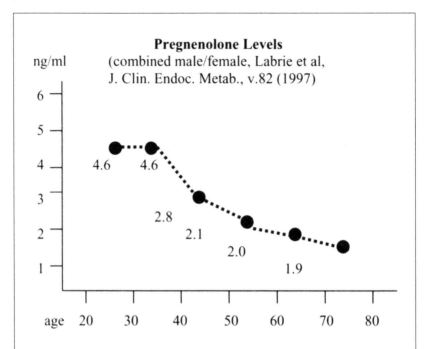

FIGURE 8.3. Pregnenolone Levels Throughout Life. This figure indicates how our pregnenolone levels fall as the body ages. Note that pregnenolone levels drop quickly starting around the age of thirty-five, and are usually only half what they were at their peak by the age of forty-five.

of fourteen different hormones in men with prostate cancer and compared them to the hormone levels of healthy men. They discovered that pregnenolone (and DHEA) levels were generally lower in the prostate cancer patients.

DOSAGE: A good dose of pregnenolone for those over forty is 50 mg a day for men and 25 mg a day for women. Do not exceed these doses.

HUMAN GROWTH HORMONE

Human growth hormone (HGH) levels fall as we age, and as they fall, the possibility of developing prostate cancer increases. Raising your HGH levels will strengthen your immunity and allow you to live a longer and better life. At the University of Naples Federico II in Italy (the *Journal of Clinical Endocrinology & Metabolism* v 88, 2003), a case-control study was done on the effects of falling HGH levels on prostate health. Researchers stated, "In conclusion, GH replacement restores prostate size to normal in both young and elderly patients with no increase in prostate abnormalities." Real human growth hormone (rHGH) costs about $3,600 a year and must be injected subcutaneously. Just because real HGH is so expensive does not mean it is a "miracle hormone"—it is expensive because the pharmaceutical corporations have colluded to make it so. Veterinary growth hormones are just as costly to produce but are sold to farmers at very economical rates. The inexpensive Chinese HGH is no longer available. There are lots of products on the market that claim to raise HGH levels, but be careful because many of these are often ineffective; "homeopathic HGH," for example, doesn't even contain HGH at all. Do not fall for these well-done promotions, no matter how enticing they sound. None of them work, no matter how well the ads are written. You can maintain a youthful level of the human growth hormone by eating a low-calorie diet, exercising regularly, staying slim, fasting, and avoiding bad habits like smoking. There are currently no saliva test kits for HGH because HGH levels must be measured by multiple blood draws; moreover, it is difficult to accurately measure HGH because blood levels may vary quite a bit during the day. Go by the real world results you get.

Note that insulin-like growth factor 1 (IGF-1, a hormone that is similar in molecular structure to insulin) levels do not parallel HGH levels, despite the conventional wisdom. High IGF-1 levels are often associated with prostate disease. Don't even consider HGH until all your other basic hormones are balanced.

DOSAGE: HGH supplements are very overrated because they are expensive, and only those over fifty who have balanced all their other basic hormones should even consider supplementing their diets with HGH. You can "spike" (but not consistently raise) your HGH levels by taking 1 g of L-glutamine in the A.M. and 1 g in the P.M., daily.

TRIIODOTHYRONINE AND THYROXINE

Prostate disease is often associated with thyroid dysfunction (the *Journal of Urology* v 168, 2002 and *Prostate Cancer* v 4, 2001). You should test both of your free (unbound, or not connected to carrier proteins like most thyroid hormones) thyroid hormone levels since all of our hormones work together, in concert, as a unified system. It is better to test your free triiodothyronine (free T_3) and free L-thyroxine (free T_4) instead of your thyroid stimulating hormone (TSH) or T_3 uptake, as your doctor might suggest. There are no saliva tests for free T_3 and free T_4 now, but there will be soon.

DOSAGE: You should only take T_3 and T_4 supplements if you have a thyroid deficiency. Pharmaceutical T_4 (Synthroid, Levoxyl, etc.) and T_3 (Cytomel, Cynomel, etc.) are bioidentical in every way. Treat your T_3 and T_4 levels completely separately and do not use Armour Thyroid® unless both your T_3 and T_4 levels are equally low; Armour® pig extract contains both T_3 and T_4 in a four to one ratio and can only be used by about 5 percent of those who are hypothyroid.

INSULIN

High insulin levels have been positively correlated with BPH as well as cancer (the *Journal of Urology* v 168, 2002, *Recent Results in Cancer Research* v 166, 2005, and the *Journal of the National Cancer Institute* v 95, 2003). High insulin levels are due to "insulin resistance," which is when your body's cells cannot properly respond when insulin tries to transport glucose from the bloodstream into the muscle tissues. Insulin resistance is another cause of prostate disease (*Hormone and Metabolic Research* v 35, 2003), and the only way you can diagnose this is by taking a glucose tolerance test (GTT). You simply drink a small cup of glucose solution, wait one hour, and test your blood sugar level. A GTT is an inexpensive test that everyone over forty should take. Your GTT result should be about 100 (and not about 110 as the medical profession claims). Your fasting blood glucose should be 85 or less (not 100 or less). Insulin resistance (and diabetes) can be cured with a wholegrain-based diet (that avoids sugars, including honey, fruit, and fruit juice as much as possible), proper supplements, hormone balancing, and exercise.

DOSAGE: As long as you maintain a healthy, low-sugar diet and test your insulin levels regularly, you should not need to take insulin supplements.

CORTISOL

Cortisol is produced by the adrenal gland, and it is released when the body responds to stress; its primary functions are to suppress the immune system, increase blood sugar, and regulate the metabolism. Cortisol is best measured with a saliva test, and since levels vary so much during the day, it is better to obtain a daily profile by measuring levels at 9:00 A.M., 1:00 P.M., 5:00 P.M., and 9:00 P.M. Most people, however, do not need to take cortisol supplements.

DOSAGE: Only diet and lifestyle are going to lower high levels of cortisol. Cortef® cortisol tablets are available, however, for those who have low levels.

THYMUS HORMONES

Surprisingly, the thymus gland and the hormones it secretes are not well understood. The thymus does not just secrete one or two simple hormones that we could easily use as supplements. As we age, this important gland involutes, or curls in on itself, until it all but disappears by the time we are forty. Obviously, this has a lot to do with aging and illness.

DOSAGE: Unfortunately, you cannot simply take thymus hormones or take thymus extracts. We need more research to be done on how to rejuvenate thymus activity as we age.

CONCLUSION

The hormones discussed throughout this chapter are all necessary in order for your body to function properly. It is particularly important for men with prostate disease to maintain healthy hormone levels. While androgens like testosterone and DHEA are especially vital to prostate health, each of the basic hormones provides significant health benefits to your prostate. Remember to regularly test your hormone levels so that you can maintain a healthy hormone balance.

9. Testosterone Is Your Friend

Nearly every medical doctor in the world will tell you that testosterone is somehow "bad" for your prostate and makes prostate cancer grow—this has become an unquestionable sacred dogma for doctors, even though the fall in testosterone as men age almost exactly parallels the rise in prostatitis, BPH, and prostate cancer. This insanity began more than eighty years ago, even before Charles Huggins got the brilliant idea to use castration as a cure for prostate cancer! Once a man has been castrated, his prostate reduces in size, so, at the time, doctors must have thought shrinking the size of the prostate—by any means possible—seemed like a good idea. The patients temporarily appeared to get better, but the cancer soon returned with a vengeance, and they quickly died. Anyone who thinks you can cure cancer by cutting off a man's testicles is sorely mistaken. This butchery has continued to the present day, however, and now doctors can use both chemicals and scalpels to castrate men.

There are over 200 published studies from clinics around the world proving beyond any doubt that testosterone helps prevent and cure all prostate disease. In this chapter, there are thirty published studies that all prove empirically that testosterone is healthy for the prostate. Every year more such studies are published, yet doctors still chemically and physically castrate men in order to reduce their testosterone levels to zero.

THE HISTORY OF TESTOSTERONE

A study on testosterone from Oxford University was published in the *Proceedings of the Royal Society of Medicine* in 1936. Testosterone was only discovered and synthesized in 1935, so it was barely known to doctors, much less available. Ironically, seventy years ago the doctors knew that estrogen was bad for prostate health and testosterone was good for prostate health; they also were aware of the all-important testosterone-to-estrogen ratio, in which testosterone should control and limit the "female hormone." Over eighty studies were quoted in the published analysis.

Another study from Louisiana State University was published in the *Journal of Urology* in 1938. In this case, the doctors understood that testosterone levels fall as men age, and the incidence of prostate disease rises greatly. Since testosterone had only been very recently discovered, the patients were given fresh animal testes with good results. The researchers referred to other studies that used extracts from animal testes as well as the recently synthesized testosterone propionate. The medical profession inherently knew that "the male hormone" was good for curing BPH, a common malady even then.

THE SCIENCE BEHIND TESTOSTERONE

As you can clearly see from Figure 9.1, Male Estrogen and Testosterone Blood Levels Throughout Life, testosterone levels fall as men age while estrogen levels rise. Testosterone dominance and the testosterone-to-estrogen ratio are reversed, and the probability of developing prostate disease increases accordingly. Remember: Common sense tells you that testosterone is your friend, has always been your friend, and will always be your friend.

The scientific literature is full of countless studies that prove testosterone is necessary for a healthy prostate and metabolism. When free testosterone levels in the blood are low, prostate receptors must choose dihydrotestosterone (DHT) instead, but DHT binding to the prostate receptors is a basic cause of illness. (Serum DHT is unrelated to prostate illness.) Let's take just some of the many dozens of published clinical studies from around the world to prove that high, youthful levels of the androgens testosterone, androstenedione, and DHEA protect you from prostate illness. Supplementing low testosterone and androgen levels will help you cure your illness. Every month more such studies are published in the international medical literature.

At the University of Washington[1] a progressive, innovative, and pioneering doctor named Richmond Prehn actually said that we should consider using androgen supplementation to reduce the growth of prostate cancer! He pointed out that declining testosterone levels contribute to carcinogenesis, and that

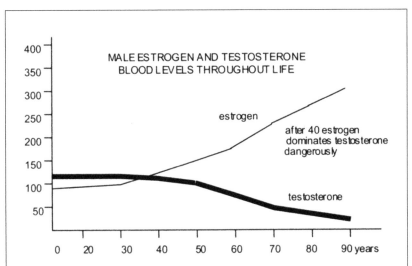

FIGURE 9.1. Male Estrogen and Testosterone Blood Levels Throughout Life. This figure depicts the average man's estrogen and testosterone levels throughout his life. Note that during his youth, a man's testosterone levels will be higher than his estrogen levels. But after he turns thirty, his testosterone-to-estrogen ratio begins to reverse, and estrogen dominates testosterone; this reversal can be very dangerous to men's health.

Adapted from *Acta Endrocrinologica* v 74, 1973 and v 80, 1970.

supplementing these low levels would reduce cancer rates. He referred to earlier studies that showed low testosterone levels in prostate cancer patients indicated a much worse prognosis. It is doctors like him that are going to lead us into the medical Age of Enlightenment, and out of the Age of Darkness.

At the University of Witwaterstrand in Africa[2] researchers conducted a study titled, "Low Serum Testosterone Predicts a Poor Outcome in Meta-static Prostate Cancer." They studied 122 patients and found that the ones with the highest testosterone levels had the least aggressive tumors, and lived the longest. The patients with the lowest testosterone levels had far more aggressive growths, and died much sooner. The doctors concluded, "Low testosterone seems to result in a more aggressive disease and a poorer prognosis in advanced prostate cancer." This study is very clear.

At the Hubei Medical University in China[3] doctors studied men with BPH and carcinoma and discovered, "The results showed that serum testosterone in patients with BPH and PCA [prostate cancer antigen] was lower than that of the healthy control group," and further, ". . . the ratio of testosterone-to-estradiol is decreased with the rise of the age. The results suggested that the imbalance of serum sex hormones (i.e., falling testosterone and rising estrogen) was related to the pathogenesis of BPH and PCA." It is low testosterone and high estrogen levels that cause prostate problems.

At Harvard Medical School[4] doctors carried out a study titled, "Is Low Serum Testosterone a Marker for High Grade Prostate Cancer?" They found that men with lower testosterone levels had more aggressive tumors, higher Gleason scores, and shorter life spans. (Gleason scores are a measure of cancer severity.) The conclusion: "In our study, patients with prostate cancer and a low free testosterone [level] had more extensive disease. In addition, all men with a biopsy Gleason score of 8 or greater had low serum free testosterone. This finding suggests that low serum free testosterone may be a marker for more aggressive disease." Again, the lower the testosterone, the worse the prognosis. Men, this is directly from Harvard Medical School.

At the University of Vienna[5] men with prostate cancer were studied for their serum testosterone levels. The doctors concluded, "Low serum testosterone in men with newly diagnosed prostate cancer is associated with higher tumor microvessel and androgen receptor density (note: both of these make the malignancies grow faster), as well as higher Gleason score, suggesting enhanced malignant potential." In other words, in men with low testosterone, the tumors grew faster, the cancer was more aggressive, and the patients died sooner.

Another study from the University of Vienna[6] was titled, "High Grade Prostate Cancer is Associated With Low Serum Testosterone Levels." These researchers found that "patients with high Gleason score prostate cancer have lower testosterone levels." The men with the lowest Gleason scores and slowest growing malignancies had high testosterone levels averaging 4.1 ng/ml; those with the highest Gleason scores and fastest growing malignancies had low testosterone levels averaging only 2.8 ng/ml. The men with almost 50 percent higher testosterone levels fared much better.

In another study at Harvard Medical School[7] doctors found that the cancer patients with the highest levels of testosterone fared the best, and lived the longest. "A high prevalence of biopsy detectable prostate cancer was identified in men with low total or free testosterone," they said. Furthermore, "A low serum testosterone level in men is associated with a number of medical conditions, most notably sexual dysfunction, and is commonly treated with exogenous (externally provided) testosterone supplementation."

At the Memphis Veterans Administration Hospital[8] doctors determined that elderly veterans fared much better when they had higher testosterone levels. "Patients with a pretreatment testosterone level of less than 300 ng/100 ml had shorter intervals free of progression than patients with pretreatment testosterone levels of greater than 300 ng/100 ml." The doctors referred to studies conducted as early as 1971 that showed the same previous phenomenon. The higher their testosterone levels, the longer the men lived; the lower their levels, the sooner they died.

In an impressive collective effort between six international clinics,[9] including the University of California at Los Angeles and Columbia University, scientists used the Norwegian Cancer Registry to study the frozen blood serum and medical records of approximately 28,000 men. The median age of the men at blood draw was sixty years old. The scientists found that the healthy men actually had higher testosterone levels than the ones who developed prostate cancer, and so they concluded that the idea of testosterone increasing the risk of prostate cancer is completely unsupported in any way. Men, this study is the second largest ever done on testosterone and prostate cancer. You just can't argue with its conclusions based on 28,000 real men.

Moreover, the University of Chicago and three other clinics[10] found the exact same results. "A separate analysis of serum testosterone levels revealed that the higher the pretreatment serum testosterone level, the greater the survival rate. Compared with patients with serum testosterone levels of less than 6.9 nmo/L, significant differences in survival were observed for patients with serum testosterone levels of 10.4 to 13.9, 13.9 to 17.3, and those higher than 17.3 nmo/L." This means that the higher the testosterone levels were, the longer the men lived, and the better they fared. "These results have important implications for the design and analysis of future clinical trials of hormone therapy." Doctors should be giving men testosterone therapy, rather than androgen ablation.

At Johns Hopkins University in Baltimore[11] more men were studied. One group was healthy, one had BPH, and one had prostate cancer. Their total testosterone (measured in ng/dl) was measured over a five-year period. The healthy men had an average level of 636.1, the BPH group only 527.4, the men with localized cancer averaged only 472.6, and those with metastatic cancer 567.7. Clearly, the healthy men had much higher levels of testosterone. Strangely enough, the conclusion was, "These data suggest that there are no measurable differences in serum testosterone levels among men who are destined to develop prostate cancer and those without the disease." These doctors simply did not want to admit that low testosterone was found in the BPH, low cancer, and metastasized cancer patients. A dramatic difference of 35 percent certainly should have proved the case decisively. They actually tried to deny their own results.

At the University of Utah[12] researchers carried out a unique study in which they compared 214 sets of male twins. Using identical twins is a most effective means to demonstrate scientific validity. The researchers found that the higher the testosterone levels, the smaller the men's prostate glands were. "Prostate volumes correlated inversely with age-adjusted serum testosterone." The men with the smallest prostates had testosterone levels of 17.7 / 7.9 / 17.9 nmo/L, while the men with the largest glands had levels of only 14.7 / 6.0 / 14.2. To prevent or cure BPH, a man certainly wants to maintain a youthful testosterone level. Any man over the age of forty should know his free testosterone levels, and supplement them as necessary.

At the Petrov Institute of Oncology in Russia,[13] men (average age about forty) were divided into two groups of high and low blood testosterone. The first group was given 120 mg daily of oral testosterone undecanoate, and the second 80 mg. In the end, the men's prostates reduced in volume, generally in six months. "These findings suggest that exogenous testosterone in middle-aged and older men with some clinical features of age-related androgen deficiency can retard or reverse prostate growth." Everyone knows that the gradual decrease in male testosterone levels after the age of thirty clearly coincides with the abnormal increase in prostate volumes (BPH). The need for testosterone supplementation is obvious, yet doctors somehow can't see this. Using oral testosterone salts was a very bad idea, the doses were too high, and they would have gotten far better results with natural transdermal or sublingual testosterone delivering about 3 mg a day.

At the famous Tenovus Institute in Wales[14] over 200 prostate cancer patients were studied. Here again, doctors found that the men with the lowest testosterone levels had the poorest prognosis and died the soonest. "Low concentrations of testosterone in plasma at the time of diagnosis related to a poor prognosis. Patients who died within one year of diagnosis had the lowest mean plasma levels of this steroid." They went on to repeat, "The results of this study suggest that low plasma testosterone concentrations in men with prostatic carcinoma at the time of initial diagnosis is associated with a poor prognosis. The highest levels of plasma testosterone were found in those patients who subsequently survived the longest." This study was done almost twenty years ago, and was published in a major journal. Why are doctors still castrating men with scalpels and toxic chemicals to destroy their testosterone? Why aren't they giving them supplements?

At the University of Connecticut[15] doctors gave elderly, hypogonadal (low testosterone) men either transdermal testosterone (the natural and correct way) or injections of testosterone (the unnatural and wrong way), for several months. They found, "There were no ill effects on prostate size, symptoms, or prostate specific antigen [PSA] level." If they had measured more health parameters, they would have found that the men responded well overall, and got many benefits from raising their testosterone. If testosterone has negative effects (as 99.9 percent of the world's doctors believe), then these doctors would have enlarged their patients' prostates, raised their PSAs, and produced higher rates of cancer—since basically all men over seventy already have growing cancer cells in their prostates. These sacred beliefs were further disproved with the low testosterone (hypogonadal), elderly men who were given supplemental testosterone. The doctors reiterated, "No significant side effects in prostate tests or symptoms were seen in this study."

A similar study was done at the Brooke Army Medical Center in Texas[16] where older men were given injections of supplemental testosterone salts for six months. The doctors concluded, "Parenteral [injection] testosterone replacement in hypogonadal men with normal pretreatment digital rectal examination and serum PSA levels does not alter PSA or PSA velocity beyond established non-treatment norms." If testosterone causes prostate problems, obviously the men's PSA levels would have gone up dramatically. The doctors should have used natural transdermal or sublingual testosterone, but still the men generally benefited from the therapy.

A quarter of a century ago at the Granada Medical Facility,[17] men with BPH were studied and compared with healthy men of the same age group. They found that the men with BPH had a 43 percent lower testosterone level than the healthy men. The men with BPH had an average level of only 2.3 ng/ml, while the healthy men's levels averaged 4.0 ng/ml. Obviously 43 percent is a very dramatic difference, and it proves yet again that low testosterone levels cause prostate disease. "The testosterone concentration in the BPH group was significantly lower than that of the healthy control group." The authors of this study were also well aware that estradiol rises strongly in men as they age, and that estradiol supplementation causes abnormal growth in the prostate gland. This study was published twenty-five years ago in a major journal, yet it is basically ignored today.

At the Royal London Hospital[18] doctors conducted a stunning review of thirty-four studies, complete with fifty-five references. They revealed that the Huggins testosterone "dogma" has been completely unsupported by science for the last sixty years. "Yet there has so far been no conclusive evidence, despite thirty-four studies, that levels of circulating testosterone in individuals developing prostate cancer are higher than in controls." They quoted other studies: "Three overviews provided similar evidence that there is no significant difference in mean testosterone levels between patients and control." They went on to say, "Firstly, prostate cancers arising in men with low serum testosterone levels are more malignant and frequently unresponsive to hormones [e.g. estrogen]." Yet most doctors continue to walk in darkness.

At the Beth Israel Hospital in New York City[19] researchers studied men for thirteen different hormones (or their metabolites) to determine which ones contributed to the growth of their carcinomas. They found that the average cancer patient had a low testosterone level of about 350 ng/dl, compared to the healthy controls' much higher levels of about 450 ng/dl. In men under sixty-five, the difference was much more dramatic, with levels of 282 ng/dl in cancer patients compared to 434 ng/dl for the healthy controls—over 50 percent higher testosterone levels in healthy men without cancer. These researchers were very reluctant to admit what they found, however, because it contradicted their dogma.

The internationally renowned Karolinska Institute in Sweden[20] studied 2,400 cancer patients and determined that the prostate cancer patients had 8 percent lower testosterone than healthy controls. Prostate cancer is the leading cause of male cancer deaths in Sweden, due mainly to high-fat diets. The conclusion: "Testosterone levels were lower in patients with cancer than in controls." Again, we see that high, youthful testosterone levels help prevent cancer.

Twenty years ago, at the University of Helsinki[21] hormones were measured in men with BPH or prostate cancer, against healthy controls. The free testosterone levels of the BPH patients averaged only 301 pmol/L, the cancer patients just 249 pmol/L, while the healthy men had a high level of 380 pmol/L. The healthy men had low estradiol levels of only 53.5 pmol/L, while the BPH patients had a stunning 137.4 pmol/L, and the cancer patients only 83.7 pmol/L. Furthermore, the healthy men had testosterone-to-estradiol ratios of 7.1:1 (the higher, the better), while the BPH men had 2.2:1, and the cancer patients 3.0:1. Yet the poor doctors still couldn't figure out that excess estrogens cause prostate disease, while high, youthful testosterone levels prevent and cure it. None so blind as those who will not see.

At Umea University Hospital in Sweden[22] almost 3,000 men, both with and without prostate cancer, were studied for their blood androgen levels. The men with the highest levels of testosterone had the least rates of cancer, while the men with the lowest levels of testosterone had the highest rates of cancer. The doctors were stunned at the results, since they clearly started out to prove that "androgens stimulate prostate cancer in vivo and in vitro." They began with a bias against testosterone, but had to reverse themselves due to their own findings.

In another study at Harvard Medical School[23] doctors really took a big risk in going against the prevailing negative view of testosterone and prostate health. They took seventy-five men with low testosterone, twenty of whom had a precancerous condition called "prostatic intraepithelial neoplasia" or PIN, and they gave all of these men supplemental testosterone for one year, knowing that the prevailing medical opinion anticipates that those men with PIN will get outright cancer. Of course, nothing of the sort happened. The men were in much better mental and physical health after raising their testosterone levels; their prostate glands prospered by having the testosterone they needed. These doctors deserve a lot of credit for their courage.

At Taipei Veterans Hospital[24] ninety-six men with advanced metastatic prostate cancer were studied for their hormone levels, including testosterone, LH, FSH, and prolactin. The men were divided into two groups based on their testosterone levels. Group 1 had 77 percent higher testosterone levels than group 2. Group 1, which fared the best, had the highest testosterone levels. Group 2, made up of those whose cancer grew quickly, had the lowest testosterone levels. The doctors concluded, "Higher testosterone and lower LH, FSH and prolactin levels were good prognostic factors for patients with metastatic prostate cancer undergoing hormonal treatment, irrespective of tumor grading." These same doctors still insisted on using ablation therapy to destroy their patients' testosterone levels. Incredible! How can they be so blind?

Over a quarter century ago at the Tenovus Institute for Cancer Research in Wales,[25] doctors found out that low testosterone was clearly correlated with both BPH and prostate cancer. Actually, they tried to deny this fact, in spite of the blood tests they had, which just proves that the medical profession is more interested in keeping the status quo than finding the truth. The healthy men had 17 percent higher testosterone levels than the men with prostate cancer, and yet the doctors tried to claim these levels "were not significantly different." Obviously, 17 percent is very statistically significant in any such study. The men with BPH also had significantly lower testosterone levels. Unfortunately, these doctors still poisoned their patients with stilbestrol (a synthetic estrogen) to destroy all testosterone production.

At Yamagata University in Japan[26] a first-rate study was carried out on men suffering from BPH. The men with BPH had 19 percent larger prostates and 39 percent higher estradiol levels compared to healthy controls. The healthy men had 49 percent higher free testosterone levels and 46 percent higher total testosterone levels. The healthy men also had an excellent testosterone-to-estrogen ratio of .99, while the diseased men had a terrible testosterone-to-estrogen ratio of .17. Again, the authors of this study actually tried to deny that the testosterone levels were related to prostate volume, since this fact contradicted the accepted medical dogma! Truth just doesn't seem to interest them, and facts only confuse them.

At the Harvard School of Public Health and other clinics[27] men (average age seventy-two) with prostate cancer were compared to healthy men. The healthy controls had 21 percent higher testosterone levels (average 541.8 ng/ml) than the cancer patients (average 447.1 ng/ml). Sadly, the authors of this study also tried (in vain) to deny that low testosterone was clearly correlated with prostate cancer. This was a very powerful human "case-control study" headed by Harvard University, but the scientists involved were so biased that they tried to deny their own data. It is such a shame that medical professionals such as these appear to be more interested in dogma and tradition than in truth and facts.

At Helsinki University in Finland,[28] 123 men (average age of seventy-two) with prostate cancer were studied for their hormone levels. The researchers concluded, "Low pretreatment values (of testosterone) indicated poorer prognosis." The lower the free testosterone levels, the higher the Gleason score. The lower the free testosterone, the more aggressive were the tumors. The lower the free testosterone, the more the cancer metastasized. After four years 80 percent of the men with the higher testosterone levels were still alive, but only 45 percent of the men with the lower testosterone levels were still alive. High testosterone levels win again.

CONCLUSION

We could go on with dozens more studies on the benefits of testosterone, but thirty should be enough to show just how strong and comprehensive the evidence behind testosterone really is. Every year, researchers around the world conduct further studies, proving again and again that testosterone is not only beneficial but also necessary for a healthy prostate.

10. Estrogens

Men and women have exactly the same hormones, only in different amounts. There is no "estrogen" per se; estrogen is merely a convenient term to use when referring to the class of hormones collectively known as estrogens. Men have smaller amounts of estrogen than women until the age of fifty, when male levels begin to rise. Female levels fall after menopause. So, middle-aged men commonly have more estrogen than women! As men's testosterone-to-estrogen ratios become reversed, the changes in their hormone levels can have very dangerous effects on their health. The reversal of this ratio is a major key to understanding not only prostate disease, but many other male illnesses, including cardiovascular health, low immunity, gynecomastia (male breast growth), abdominal fat, baldness, and various cancers.

THE TRUTH ABOUT ESTROGENS

There are actually three basic estrogens: estradiol or E_2 (the most powerful and most carcinogenic); estrone or E_1; and estriol or E_3 (the weakest, safest, and most beneficial estrogen). Estradiol and estrone comprise about 20 percent of human estrogen, and estriol about 80 percent. (Men rarely have any estriol imbalance and do not need to test their estriol levels as women do.) The testosterone-to-estrogen ratio reversal that occurs as we age creates high levels of estradiol and estrone in men. Unfortunately, high estradiol and estrone levels cause prostate disease.

the science behind the testosterone-to-estrogen ratio

Over the last forty years there have been dozens of studies showing the harmful effect of excessive estrogen in aging males caused by the reversed androgen-to-estrogen ratio (including androstenedione and DHEA, in addition to testosterone). It is beyond the scope of this book, and would likely bore the reader, to list and discuss the dozens of studies. We will pick twenty of them to quickly prove that testosterone is your friend, and excess estrogen is your enemy. The reversal of the androgen-to-estrogen ratio is the most important insight we have into prostate disease.

At the University of Hamburg (*Prostate* v 3, 1982) doctors found high levels of estrogens in men with prostate enlargement. "In conclusion, there is a distinct accumulation of estrogens in the nuclei of stroma, estradiol concentration being significantly higher—thus stimulating the growth of BPH." Excessive estradiol and estrone are the main biochemical cause of prostate disease. In a second study performed at the same university (the *Journal of Steroid Biochemistry and Molecular Biology* v 19, 1983), men with BPH were found to have (a) excessive estradiol in their prostates, (b) high 5-alpha-reductase activity, and (c) increased DHT accumulation.

At the Bielanski Hospital in Poland (Roczniki Akademii Medicina v 42, 1984) men with prostate cancer generally had high serum estradiol and low serum testosterone, displaying the classic testosterone-to-estrogen ratio reversal. At the American Health Foundation in New York (Prostate v 5, 1984) doctors discovered that "persons with prostate cancer had higher estrone and estradiol levels in prostatic fluid." At TNB College in India (the *Indian Journal of Physiology and Pharmacology* v 29, 1985) scientists studied men with BPH and determined that the patients had high estrone levels in their prostate glands, but had low pregnenolone levels. At the Sloan-Kettering Institute (Prostate v 9, 1986) researchers found high levels of estrogens in BPH patients. "Total estrogens produced in BPH patients was 223 fmol/mg compared with healthy controls with only 102 fmol/mg." Likewise, at the University of Miami (Prostate v 21, 1992) doctors found high estrogens in men with BPH; they concluded that "local estrogen production in the stroma and/or epithelium of the prostate plays a role in the . . . development of BPH."

At Schering AG in Berlin (the *Journal of Steroid Biochemistry and Molecular Biology* v 44, 1993) doctors recommended, "Consequently, estrogen deprivation might be a new, useful principle for a conservative treatment of BPH." At Ruhr University Bochum in Germany (the *Journal of Clinical Endocrinology and Metabolism* v 77, 1993) doctors said, " . . . the prostatic accumulation of DHT, estradiol, and estrone is intimately correlated with aging, leading to the increase of the estrogen/testosterone ratio in BPH." Like their colleagues from other studies, these doctors also found higher estradiol and estrone levels in the glands of their BPH patients.

At the University of Bonn (the *Journal of Steroid Biochemistry and Molecular Biology* v 44, 1993), wise doctors used estrogen blockers to lower estradiol and estrone in BPH patients with dramatic results. Serum estrogen levels fell strongly. Prostate volumes fell from 74.2 to 64.0 in only ninety days. The doctors strongly recommended estrogen deprivation for BPH. Using suicide substrate aromatase inhibitors such as 1,4,6-Androstatriene-3,17-dione (ATD)—which blocks the synthesis of estrogens—is infinitely better than taking toxic drugs such as atamestane. At Harvard Medical School (the *Journal of Clinical Endocrinology and Metabolism* v 77, 1993) 320 men with BPH were compared to 320 healthy men. High plasma estradiol levels were clearly related to BPH, as well as to the obviously reversed testosterone-to-estrogen ratio. And low androgen levels were clearly related to BPH. Studies like these are groundbreaking, even though they took place almost twenty years ago.

At Gunma University in Japan (the *Scandinavian Journal of Urology and Nephrology* v 29, 1995), doctors stated that " . . . an estrogen dominated environment plays an important role in the development of BPH." Specifically, they determined that estrogen levels unmistakably correlated to prostate volumes.

At the University of Vienna (*Wiener Klinische Woschenschrift* v 110, 1998) twenty-three clinical trials, spanning fifteen years, were reviewed. The researchers found that estrogen (not testosterone) suppression was the proper treatment for BPH. "The estrogen suppression . . . is considered as an efficient pharmacotherapeutic strategy in the medical treatment of uncomplicated BPH." If these good doctors had reached a little further, they might have realized that testosterone supplementation is the next step.

In another study at Gunma University (*Prostate* v 42, 2000), doctors found high estradiol in BPH patients. A different group of doctors at Yamagata University came across similar results (the *Journal of Urology* v 21, 2000): "Serum estradiol levels correlating with the prostate volume, whereas free testosterone levels did not." Still more Japanese doctors (*Rinsho Byori* v 52, 2004) determined, "Estrogen may play a pathophysiological role in BPH . . . due to increased estrogen and decreased testosterone. Estrogen plays a physiological role in BPH." Back in the United States, the doctors at Northwestern University (*Prostate* v 41, 1999) came to the same conclusion. Estrogen dominates testosterone after a man reaches the age of fifty, and this hormonal trend is a major cause of prostate growth.

A 2007 review of the scientific literature (the *Journal of Cellular Biochemistry* v 102) clearly indicated that high levels of estrogen are the endocrinological cause of prostate disorders. The researchers concluded, "Multiple, consistent evidence suggests that estrogens are critical players in human prostate cancer, their role was only recently considered, being eclipsed for years by an androgen-dominated interest." Furthermore, a slightly more recent review (the *European Journal of Cancer* v 44, 2008) stated, "This leads to the intriguing notion that estradiol may be the initiating driver of prostate cancer . . . anti-estrogens might be an overlooked treatment."

Another study published the very same year (the *Journal of Steroid Biochemistry and Molecular Biology* v 109, 2008) found estrone to be "significantly higher in prostate cancer." Yet another study from 2008 (the Journal of Endocrinology v 197, 2008) stated, "Estrogens have been implicated as a cause of BPH. These findings support the hypothesis that estrogen plays a role in the pathogenesis of BPH."

A recent study (the *European Journal of Cancer Prevention* v 19, 2010) found high estrogens in prostate cancer. "The action of unopposed estrogen directly initiates, promotes, and exacerbates prostatic enlargement and prostate cancer. This controversial breakthrough represents a paradigm shift in medical thinking, which can prevent the raging pandemic of cancer sweeping the world." The doctors also found unopposed estrogen to be the base cause of obesity, diabetes, and breast cancer. In a different study from 2010 (*Urology* v 76, 2010), the researchers clearly stated, "In this cohort of older men, higher estrone levels were strongly associated with increased risk of incident prostate cancer."

For decades, researchers and scientists have revealed the prostate health benefits of testosterone, along with the dangers of estrogens. Note that there is also overwhelming evidence from animal studies (which date back over forty years) that proves that the estrogens estradiol and estrone are basic contributors to BPH, prostatitis, and cancer. Of course, scientists should conduct more human studies, and finally these are being started. Indeed, even the most recent clinical trials on the subject indicate that high estrogen levels in men help cause prostate disease.

CONCLUSION

High estradiol and estrone levels are the real cause of prostate disease. Unfortunately, it is difficult to lower estrogen levels. The current prescription estrogen blockers and aromatase inhibitors are very toxic, dangerous, and have serious side effects. Aromatase is the enzyme that converts testosterone to estradiol, and androstene-dione to estrone. It is very difficult to lower aromatase or to prevent aromatase activity (except by implementing the diet, exercise, and lifestyle changes described in earlier chapters, as well as taking proven supplements such as DIM and flax oil). Sadly, the suicide substrate aromatase inhibitors like ATD are not available over the counter, or even by prescription.

Remember, you can only lower estrogen levels by eating a low-fat diet, consuming fewer calories, and exercising regularly. You should also take DIM and flax oil to raise your testosterone, androstenedione, and DHEA levels. It is especially critical to avoid eating saturated animal fats. Consuming saturated animal fats and being overweight are the two biggest causes of elevated estradiol and estrone levels. The most important factor here is maintaining a low-fat diet.

11. Home Hormone Testing

Prostate conditions are largely hormone-based. Our prostates are more affected by hormones than any other factor. Ironically, even urologists almost never test their patients' hormone levels, especially testosterone. If you were to demand a hormone test from your doctor, it would require getting blood drawn, paying up to $100 per hormone tested, going on a second office visit, and then usually purchasing for an expensive prescription. The test results that come back to you often do not distinguish between bound (unavailable levels) and free (bioavailable levels). Ranges can be vague, and most doctors do not know the difference between bound and unbound hormones. In fact, most doctors are simply unaware of which hormones to test, how to test them, and how to administer supplemental ones. Even endocrinologists are surprisingly uninformed about hormone testing and administration, though this is their specialty. Unfortunately, most naturopaths, holistic doctors, and life extension specialists are equally ignorant. Which means: It is left up to you to test your hormone levels and maintain a healthy balance.

UNDERSTANDING HOW HOME HORMONE TESTING WORKS

Proteins in our bloodstream called sex hormone-binding globulins (SHBG) bind themselves to the majority of our sex hormones, making them biologically unavailable. Testosterone, for example, is about 98 percent bound. This leaves only about 2 percent free, bioavailable testosterone that actually affects our metabolic processes. Only your free, unbound hormone levels matter.

For over twenty years now, scientists have been able to accurately measure hormone levels by using saliva samples. Previously, this has taken place only in clinics and medical studies. Now, with technological advances, saliva samples can be collected at home, and sent to a laboratory for a radioimmunoassay (RIA) analysis. All this can be achieved at a cost of less than $30 per hormone. The World Health Organization approved this method of hormone testing in the 1990s due to its ease, efficiency, reliability, and practicality. Now you can test estradiol, estrone, estriol, testosterone, DHEA, melatonin, pregnenolone, androstenedione, cortisol, and other hormones by simply putting your saliva into a test tube and mailing it to one of several testing labs. (Progesterone is best tested with a serum blood draw as it is fat-soluble.) Soon, we'll also be able to saliva test insulin, our T_3 and T_4 thyroid hormones, as well as the human growth hormone. Though some states, including California and New York, ban home hormone testing in order to protect the medical profession's monopoly.

Saliva testing is a tremendous breakthrough in both traditional medicine and alternative, natural medicine. Very few people are aware of it, and even fewer know where to buy the test kits. You would think these kits would be available in every pharmacy and drugstore. It may take years for such a great advance in diagnostic medicine to become widely utilized.

MEASURING AND BALANCING THE LEVELS OF YOUR BASIC HORMONES

No matter what illness you are suffering from, remember that doctors of any kind rarely test your basic hormones. Ideally, you would have a complete scan of your twelve major male hormones. Obviously, your hormones are extremely critical to every aspect of your health, including mental functioning. Young people who are ill should have their basic hormones tested, and everyone over the age of forty definitely needs to know the levels of their basic hormones. You will never enjoy good health and long life unless your endocrine system is balanced at youthful levels.

It is a little-known fact that men and women have exactly the same hormones, only in different amounts. Women have the androgens DHEA, testosterone, and androstenedione. And men have progesterone, prolactin (the milk secreting hormone), luteinizing hormone (LH), follicle-stimulating hormone (FSH), and the three basic estrogens. Women even have a prostate specific antigen (PSA), and yet they have no prostate gland! The vast majority of people have no idea what any of their vital hormone levels are, or whether they are too high or too low. You can never know the true state of your health, or obtain your optimum health, unless you know your basic hormone levels and balance them to youthful ranges. It would be ideal to achieve the levels you had at age thirty. Youthful levels are your goal.

Testosterone

Over 90 percent of men over the age of fifty have low testosterone and need supplementation. Refer to Figure 11.1, Salivary Testosterone Levels Throughout Life, to see how testosterone levels in our saliva fall significantly as we age. Measure your free (not bound) testosterone. You can improve your testosterone levels by using .5 g of a 3-percent transdermal cream. Or you can take 4 mg sublingual testosterone enathate in vegetable oil (but free testosterone tastes terrible); this will give you 3 mg of actual free testosterone. You can make your own Dimethyl sulfoxide (DMSO) solution and use 3 mg of free testosterone or 4 mg of testosterone enanthate. Take your testosterone supplement only in the morning, and never use oral forms, injections, patches, weak gels, or steroids. Watch out for estrogen spillover and androgen resistance. These conditions will result in high estradiol and estrone levels, but low testosterone levels. If you suffer from either, how-

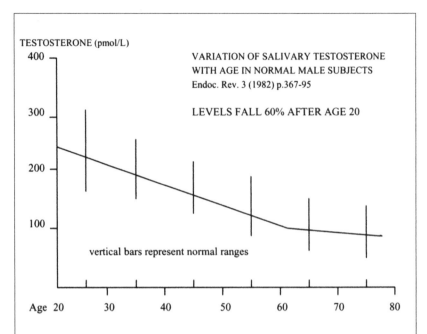

FIGURE 11.1. Salivary Testosterone Levels Throughout Life. This figure illustrates how your salivary testosterone levels fall as you age. By measuring your salivary testosterone levels with saliva test kits, you can determine whether or not you need testosterone supplements. Salivary levels peak around age twenty but fall 60 percent from then on, so 90 percent of men over the age of fifty can and should benefit from proper testosterone supplements.

ever, you can use "suicide substrate aromatase inhibitors" like ATD. These substances block the aromatase enzyme and allow your endogenous testosterone levels to rise, and your estrogens to fall. ATD is twenty times stronger than 3,6,17-androstenetrione (6-OXO), the other leading suicide substrate aromatase inhibitor. These supplements are just inexpensive analogs of androstenedione, but unfortunately, they are not available by prescription.

Dehydroepiandrosterone

Measure your free DHEA or DHEA-S (sulfate) levels. Again, you want the youthful level you had at age thirty. If your levels are low, you can take 25 mg of oral DHEA. DHEA is called the "life extension hormone" for good reason. If your DHEA is too high, only diet and lifestyle will lower it. If taking DHEA causes a rise in estradiol or estrone, then you are androgen resistant and may need to use suicide substrate aromatase inhibitors.

Estrogens

As we discussed in the previous chapter, there are three major estrogens. As men age, their estradiol and estrone levels rise, while their testosterone levels falls. This reverses the traditional testosterone-to-estrogen ratio, and causes serious problems, such as prostate disease, breast enlargement, baldness, weight gain, heart problems, and many other conditions. (Estriol is rarely out of line in men.) Test your free (not bound) estradiol and estrone levels with a saliva test kit. You want low levels ideally, and you can use the postmenopausal female levels for your range. This test is very important, since these two estrogens are the basic internal cause of prostate disease. If your levels are normal, or higher, then lower them with diet and lifestyle. Do not use toxic prescription anti-aromatase or estrogen-blocker drugs.

Progesterone

We have seen already how important progesterone is. Ideally this should be measured by a serum (not plasma) blood draw, as it is fat-soluble. It does not test well by saliva, and actually, you really don't need to test your progesterone levels. Just use $\frac{1}{8}$ teaspoon of a good transdermal cream five days a week. You can apply this to thin skin like that on your inner wrist, or directly to your scrotum for even better results. Progesterone is safe and nontoxic, so you don't have to worry about taking too much with a mere $\frac{1}{8}$ teaspoon, and only five days a week at that.

Cortisol

Using a four sample (9/1/5/9) profile to measure your cortisol levels is best. Cortisol can go up and down radically during the day and night. The truth is you really don't need to test your cortisol levels at all. Cortisol is what it is. Only diet and lifestyle will raise or lower your levels effectively. If you have very low cortisol levels, however, you can take 5 mg Cortef® tablets at the exact time of day you are low, but this is not very practical. Diet and lifestyle will normalize your levels.

Insulin

Your fasting blood sugar level should be 85 or less. Remember that magic number: 85 or less. If you cannot achieve low levels, however, get a one-hour glucose tolerance test (GTT) to determine possible insulin resistance. Look for a result of 10 mg/dl less than the accepted standard. You can also buy glycated hemoglobin (HbA1c) kits inexpensively at the drugstore; these give you a six-month average of your blood sugar levels. High blood sugar and insulin resistance is epidemic in America. Now we know these contribute to prostate disease, so keep your blood sugar and insulin low.

Human Growth Hormone

Human Growth hormone (HGH) falls dramatically as we age. This is a very overrated and expensive hormone. It will cost $1,200 to $2,400 a year for 1 IU daily, and should be injected. HGH levels vary radically during the day, especially when you are asleep. If you want to test your HGH levels, you must go to a specialty clinic and get a twelve-hour profile. IGF-1 levels do not parallel HGH levels, despite the common wisdom. In fact, men with prostate disease usually have high IGF-1 levels. If you are over fifty and want to use HGH, just go by actual physical, measurable benefits achieved after ninety days. As discussed earlier, diet and lifestyle will keep your HGH levels up. None of the over-the-counter supplements have any legitimacy at all, regardless of their impressive claims. You must use real prescription HGH daily by injection. Sublingual use in DMSO works, but doctors cannot prescribe this form; the molecule is too large to use with DMSO for regular transdermal use. The HGH molecule chain is very long (191 amino acids) and will not go through the skin intact. You cannot shake or shock HGH, or it will break and become useless. The bottom line: HGH is overrated simply because it is very expensive. If you are over fifty, balance all your other hormones before even considering HGH therapy.

Melatonin

Melatonin has to be ordered separately, as it must be collected by itself at 3:00 A.M. in the morning. If you are over forty you can generally safely take 3 mg of melatonin at night without first testing your levels. A few companies do offer melatonin saliva kits, and it is obviously not realistic to go to a sleep clinic in the middle of the night to measure your melatonin levels.

Pregnenolone

It is not easy to find pregnenolone saliva testing kits for some reason. If you are over forty, you can generally safely take 50 mg. You can see a doctor and get a blood test, or find an Internet blood testing service without a doctor. Soon we should have wider choice in saliva test kits for pregnenolone.

Triiodothyronine and Thyroxine

Low thyroid function is epidemic in western countries, and doctors are especially poor in diagnosing this. Just get your free Triiodothyronine (T_3) and free Thyroxine (T_4) levels measured with a blood draw. These levels must be midrange here, and not merely "in range." Low normal range is called "subclinical hypothyroidism." If the normal scale is, say, 1–3, then you want to be as close to 2 as possible. Doctors will generally tell you that you are fine if you are in range, but this is just not true. Your levels must be midrange for both free T_3 and free T_4. You don't need to be concerned with any other thyroid tests unless you have a serious problem with this gland. You can see a doctor or use one of the Internet blood testing services without a doctor. Web sites like www.HealthCheckUSA.com, for example, will test your hormone levels for under $100, no doctor necessary.

CONCLUSION

Search the Internet for "saliva hormone testing" or "saliva hormone test" to find home hormone testing kits. For blood tests, just search for "blood testing." If you do not have access to the Internet, get a relative to help you, or go to your local public library for assistance. The saliva kits just aren't sold in retail stores yet. If you live outside of the United States, you can send in the saliva kits using couriers such as UPS. Always test your hormone samples around 9:00 a.m. (except melatonin) for consistency. You should monitor the levels of all your basic hormones (that you choose to supplement) at least once a year.

Balancing your hormone levels is one of the last steps along the way to a healthy prostate. Together with a wholegrain-based diet, proven supplements, exercise, and occasional fasting, hormone balancing will greatly improve your health. And that's all there is to the natural prostate cure.

Seven Steps to Natural Health

The following steps are of vital importance if you want to live a long and healthy life. With these seven steps you can cure "incurable" illnesses like cancer, diabetes, and heart disease using natural treatments rather than dangerous prescription drugs, surgery, or chemotherapy. Do your best to follow every step, and note that there is also an optional eighth step that recommends prayer or meditation.

1. Maintain an American macrobiotic wholegrain-based diet. Diet is the most crucial factor in achieving good health. Diet cures disease. Everything else is secondary.

2. Take proven supplements to enhance the effects of your diet. There are forty-nine scientifically recommended supplements for those over forty.

3. Balance your hormone levels. The fourteen basic hormones are listed on page 82, and you can easily (and inexpensively) measure your hormone levels from the comfort of your own home.

4. Exercise regularly, even if that only means taking a thirty-minute walk every day. Exercise is vital, and it is best to have a balanced workout of aerobics and resistance training.

5. Fast one day a week, drinking only water from dinner to dinner. Fasting is the most powerful healing method known to man. Join our monthly Young Again two-day fast—the fasting calendar is at *www.YoungAgain.org* during the last weekend of every month.

6. Do not take prescription drugs, except *temporary* antibiotics or pain medication during an emergency. (Of course, there are rare exceptions. Diabetics, for example, need to take insulin.)

7. Limit or end any bad habits such as drinking alcohol or coffee, using recreational drugs, or eating desserts. You don't have to be a saint, but you do have to be sincere.

References

CHAPTER 9

1. *Cancer Research* v 59, 1999.

2. *American Journal of Clinical Oncology* v 20, 1997.

3. *Hubei Yike Daxue Xuebao* v 19, 1998.

4. *Journal of Urology* v 163, 2000.

5. *Journal of Urology* v 169, 2003.

6. *Prostate* v 47, 2001.

7. *Journal of the American Medical Association* v 276, 1996.

8. *Journal of Urology* v 144, 1989.

9. *Cancer Epidemiology, Biomarkers Preview* v 6, 1997.

10. *Journal of the American Medical Association* v 265, 1991.

11. *Prostate* v 27, 1995.

12. *Journal of Clinical Endocrinology and Metabolism* v 82, 1997.

13. *International Journal of Andrology* v 25, 2002.

14. *European Journal of Cancer* v 20, 1984.

15. *Endocrine Research* v 26, 2000.

16. *Journal of Urology* v 158, 1997.

17. *Experientia* v 35, 1978.

18. *Drugs & Aging* v 17, 2000.

19. *Prostate* v 3, 1982.

20. *British Journal of Urology* v 77, 1996.

21. *Prostate* v 4, 1983.

22. *International Journal of Cancer* v 108, 2003.

23. *Journal of Urology* v 170, 2003.

24. *British Journal of Urology International* v 89, 2002.

25. *Acta Endocrinologica* v 81, 1976.

26. *Journal of Andrology* v 21, 2000.

27. *Cancer Causes and Controls* v 8, 1997.

28. *Prostate* v 12, 1988.

About the Author

 Roger Mason is an internationally known research chemist who studies natural health and longevity. He has written ten different unique and cutting edge books about his findings. He sold Beta Prostate® in 2011, walked away from radio and TV, and formed a charitable trust. He lives with his wife and dog in Wilmington, NC, where they run Young Again Products. You can get his free weekly newsletter, read his books, and his 300 articles for free at www.youngagain.org.

Index

estrone (E$_1$), 109
human growth hormone
  (HGH), 90–92, 120
insulin, 92–93, 120
melatonin, 86–89, 121
pregnenolone, 89–90, 121
progesterone, 81–84, 119
testosterone, 95–107,
  117–118
thyroxine (T$_4$), 92, 121–122
triiodothyronine (T$_3$), 92,
  121–122
Human growth hormone
  (HGH), 90–92, 120
Hydrogenated fats, 14

I

*Indian Journal of Physiology and
  Pharmacology*, 110
Inflammation, 66–67
Insulin, 92–93, 120
Insulin resistance, 6, 9
Integrative Cancer Therapies, 5
*International Congressional
  Series*, 88
International Journal of Cancer,
  6, 8
*International Journal of
  Immunopharmacology*,
  67–68
*International Journal of
  Molecular Medicine*, 65
*International Journal of
  Thymology*, 87
Iodine, 45
Iron, 45

J

Journal of Cellular Biochemistry,
  112
*Journal of Clinical Endocrinology
  and Metabolism*, 91, 111
Journal of Pineal Research, 88
*Journal of Steroid Biochemistry
  and Molecular Biology*, 89,
  110, 111, 113
*Journal of the National Cancer
  Institute*, 16
Journal of Urology, 6, 96, 112

K

Klinische Endokrinologie, 57
Kushi, Michio, 4

L

Lancet, The, 55
L-glutamine, 31
Lipids, 17
Lipoic acid, 31–32

M

Magyar Onkologia, 86
Manganese, 46
Medizinische Klinik, 58–59
Melatonin, 86–89, 121
Milk thistle, 34–35
Minerals
  boron, 41
  calcium, 42
  cesium, 42–43
  chromium, 43

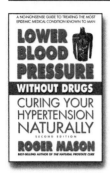

LOWER BLOOD PRESSURE
WITHOUT DRUGS, SECOND EDITION
Roger Mason

More than sixty-five million Americans have high blood pressure, which is defined as 140/90. Over forty million more are pre-hypertensive, with blood pressures reaching 120/80. High blood pressure can cause strokes, heart attacks, and congestive heart failure. Although prescription drugs may be able to lower blood pressure, they often have very dangerous side effects. The good news is that there are natural alternatives to lowering blood pressure and preventing serious disease.

In this updated edition of *Lower Blood Pressure Without Drugs,* author Roger Mason provides a uniquely nutritional approach to lowering blood pressure. The book begins by explaining hypertension—what it is, how it is diagnosed, and what causes it. It then describes how a healthy diet, rich in whole grains and low in fat, can improve both blood pressure and general health. Special chapters address important topics such as nutritional supplements, exercise, hormonal balance, and overcoming bad habits.

Be good to yourself. With this eye-opening book in hand, take the first steps towards safely and effectively lowering your blood pressure without the use of drugs.

FEBRUARY 2012 • $9.95 US • 128 pages • 6 x 9-inch quality paperback • ISBN 978-0-7570-0366-0

LOWER YOUR CHOLESTEROL
WITHOUT DRUGS, SECOND EDITION
Roger Mason

According to the American Heart Association, high cholesterol is the leading cause of coronary heart disease, which continues to be the number-one killer in North America. While millions of Americans take prescription medications to lower their cholesterol, the fact is, these drugs often have very dangerous side effects. In his updated edition of *Lower Your Cholesterol Without Drugs,* best-selling author Roger Mason offers you safe and natural alternatives to effectively lower your cholesterol levels. He does so in a no-holds barred manner, separating the fairy tales from the scientifically valid truths.

If you think it's time to achieve a healthy cholesterol level without using risky prescription drugs, you have come to the right place. Doing so is neither complicated nor expensive—it is simply a matter of knowing the simple steps to take. In *Lower Your Cholesterol Without Drugs,* you will have the solution in hand.

MARCH 2012 • $9.95 US • 128 pages • 6 x 9-inch quality paperback • ISBN 978-0-7570-0367-7

THE NATURAL DIABETES CURE
SECOND EDITION
Roger Mason

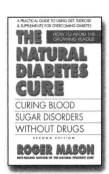

Nearly twenty million people in North America have diabetes, and each year the number continues to grow. What's most distressing is that diabetes can be easily prevented by simply maintaining a healthy balanced diet. Unfortunately, many people don't realize the serious consequences of that routine trip to their favorite fast food restaurant. Fortunately, however, best-selling author and health advocate Roger Mason is here to help with his updated edition of *The Natural Diabetes Cure*. In it, he provides a simple, yet effective nutritional approach to preventing and combating diabetes.

Divided into two parts, *The Natural Diabetes Cure* begins by explaining how diabetes develops, its major causes, and the severe health risks associated with this metabolic disorder. Part Two details how a balanced diet of whole grains, fresh fruits, vegetables, and healthy fats not only helps improve overall health and well-being, but also prevents conditions like high blood pressure, obesity, and insulin resistance, which can lead to type-2 diabetes.

Living with diabetes does not have to be a life sentence. You have the power to free yourself from this disorder. *The Natural Diabetes Cure*—with the very latest information on natural, safe, and effective treatments—will show you how.

MARCH 2012 • $9.95 US • 144 pages • 6 x 9-inch quality paperback • ISBN 978-0-7570-0369-1

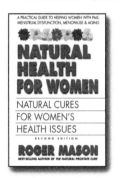

NATURAL HEALTH FOR WOMEN
SECOND EDITION
Roger Mason

Every day, millions of women are subject to their changing hormones, which play a vital role in the functioning of a healthy body. When hormones are not produced in the proper amounts or they are not in balance with one another, a number of health problems can occur, including premenstrual syndrome (PMS), pelvic inflammatory disease (PID), menstrual dysfunction, fibrocystic breasts, and menopause. Symptoms of hormonal imbalance can range from mild cramping, irritability, and food cravings to hot flashes, night sweats, and mood swings. Even serious conditions and diseases, such as osteoporosis, arthritis, diabetes, premature aging, and cancer, can result. Standard hormone replacement therapies are often used to maintain proper balance; but they can have dangerous side effects. Roger Mason, in his newly revised *Natural Health for Women*, offers safe and naturally effective alternatives to help keep hormones in balance.

Hormones do not have to control your life. With *Natural Health for Women*, you can learn to effectively maintain their proper balance safely and naturally.

MARCH 2012 • $9.95 US • 144 pages • 6 x 9-inch quality paperback • ISBN 978-0-7570-0368-4

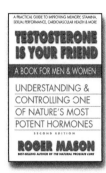

TESTOSTERONE IS YOUR FRIEND
SECOND EDITION
Roger Mason

Considered the principal male sex hormone, testosterone is responsible for stimulating and controlling characteristics that are considered "masculine," like muscles and hair growth. What many people don't realize is that this hormone is present to a lesser degree in females. What's more, low testosterone levels can cause countless health problems for both sexes, including memory loss, anxiety and depression, osteoporosis, increased cholesterol levels, weight gain, sexual dysfunction, and infertility. While testosterone supplements are available, most are ineffective and some are even dangerous.

In the updated edition of *Testosterone Is Your Friend*, author Roger Mason presents the latest and most effective natural treatments and supplements to help raise testosterone levels. The book begins by looking at how the body uses testosterone and how this hormone functions differently in men and women. Later chapters examine how testosterone deficiency affects various health conditions.

It's time to re-energize. With *Testosterone Is Your Friend,* you will have the latest information on how to increase your testosterone levels safely and naturally. By following the advice within, you can improve not only your sex life, but also the overall quality of your life.

APRIL 2012 • $9.95 US • 128 pages • 6 x 9-inch quality paperback • ISBN 978-0-7570-0371-4

ZEN MACROBIOTICS
FOR EVERYONE, SECOND EDITION
Roger Mason

In today's busy stress-filled world, maintaining a healthy, balanced diet can be a constant struggle. Making the right food choices is not always a priority. We may be considered an educated society, yet seem to be blind to the fact that our diets are typically unhealthy—low in whole grains, legumes, and fresh produce, and high in processed, fat-laden, sugary foods 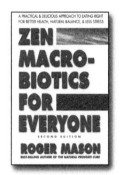 and beverages. This unwholesome diet puts us at risk for such serious health conditions as heart disease, arthritis, diabetes, and cancer. The truth is that practicing good dietary health is not as difficult or as time consuming as people might think.

A balanced diet and lifestyle can both prevent illness and serve as a powerful healer. With *Zen Macrobiotics for Everyone* in hand, you will learn the simplest and most effective ways to achieve both balance and good health in your life.

MAY 2012 • $9.95 US • 128 pages • 6 x 9-inch quality paperback • ISBN 978-0-7570-0372-1